Khedidja MESRI
Samira Rached
Aicha IDDER

Epidemiological and clinical aspects of uveal melanoma

Khedidja MESRI
Samira Rached
Aicha IDDER

Epidemiological and clinical aspects of uveal melanoma

in western Algeria

ScienciaScripts

Imprint
Any brand names and product names mentioned in this book are subject to trademark, brand or patent protection and are trademarks or registered trademarks of their respective holders. The use of brand names, product names, common names, trade names, product descriptions etc. even without a particular marking in this work is in no way to be construed to mean that such names may be regarded as unrestricted in respect of trademark and brand protection legislation and could thus be used by anyone.

Cover image: www.ingimage.com

This book is a translation from the original published under ISBN 978-620-6-70501-7.

Publisher:
Sciencia Scripts
is a trademark of
Dodo Books Indian Ocean Ltd. and OmniScriptum S.R.L publishing group

120 High Road, East Finchley, London, N2 9ED, United Kingdom
Str. Armeneasca 28/1, office 1, Chisinau MD-2012, Republic of Moldova, Europe
Printed at: see last page
ISBN: 978-620-7-68655-1

Tables of contents

CHAPTER I :
INTRODUCTION

Uveal melanoma (UM) is the most common primary intraocular tumor in adults, with a peak frequency between the ages of 55 and 65, and an annual incidence that has remained stable over the past 50 years, of the order of 5 to 9 cases per million people, with no gender predominance. It affects the Caucasian race, and is exceptional imelanoderma [1].

In Europe, the incidence of intraocular melanoma has risen since the 1970s, coinciding with an increase of more than 50% in the population aged 65 and over, and is estimated at 0.8-0.9 cases per 100,000 inhabitants/year. However, worldwide epidemiological data show an overall stable incidence compared to cutaneous melanoma [2].

Uveal melanoma is a rare cancer with a dismal prognosis, despite considerable advances in early diagnosis and quality of care in developed countries.

The clinical presentation of choroidal and ciliary body melanomas depends on a multitude of factors, principally their location in the uvea, their histopathological features and their mode of growth [3].

The main reason for consultation is reduced visual acuity, due to extension of exudative retinal detachment into the macular region, loss of transparency of the media, or tumor invasion of the macula [3].

The main method for treating intraocular melanoma, outside the indications for radical treatment, is accelerated proton beam irradiation, a technique developed in Boston in 1975, based on an idea by Robert Wilson in Berkeley in 1954. The leading centers at the time were the Massachusetts General Hospital in Boston and the Harvard cyclotron [81]. Two facilities in France treat around 600 patients a year [81].

The aim of this work is to study the epidemiological profile and clinical aspects of malignant melanoma of the choroid and ciliary body in the population of western Algeria.

Chapter II :
Epidemiology of uveal melanoma:

1. History :

The first descriptions of pigmented skin and eye tumors date back to the early 19th century.

In 1806, Laennec introduced the term "melanosis" to define the various pigmented tumors and their metastases.

In 1823, Savenko described a case of ocular melanosis, and in 1833 Bendz published in the Netherlands the first description of a choroid melanoma treated by enucleation, followed by orbital recurrence and metastases [3].

In 1863, Von Graefe published the first precise description of the clinic and pathology of melanomas, but it wasn't until 1930 that a synthesis and statistical analysis of the material collected over the last sixty years was carried out.

In 1930, Jaensh, in 1930, 1933 and 1936, Von Hippel, in 1935, Terry and Johns and, in 1936, Denecke presented the first systematic studies on vital prognosis, 5 years after enucleation. [3]

2.1   – Incidence of uveal melanoma :

Uveal melanomas are the most common primary intraocular tumors, their incidence varying from one region of the globe to another and depending on race as well as the demographic profile of the population [36], melanomas preferably affect Caucasians, and are exceptional in African, Asian and Latin American races, they are also very rare in prepubertal children [3].

Scotto et al. estimated the incidence of uveal melanoma at 0.6 cases per 100,000 inhabitants per year between 1969 and 1971 [4], but from the 1970s onwards, the incidence of melanoma in Europe increased slightly to around 0.8 to 0.9 cases per 100,000 inhabitants per year (Table 1).

The increase in melanoma incidence coincides with a rise of over 50% in the population aged over 65, the population at risk, and a reduction in the population under 20, in whom the risk is negligible, an incidence that remains stable compared to cutaneous melanomas [3].

In Saudi Arabia, 40 cases of uveal melanoma were recorded at the King Khaled Eye Specialist Hospital between 1983 and 2005, including 28 Saudi patients, and 12 patients from other Arab countries[5].

In Tunisia, at the Hédi Raies Institute in Tunis, over a 23-year period from January 1990 to December 2013, 80 cases of uveal melanoma were recorded [6]

In our department, a reference center for the western region of Algeria, a case series study over a 14-year period from 2001 to 2014, listed 30 uveal melanomas, 19 women and 11 men[1]

Authors and references	Period	Incidence	Country
Mork 1961	1953-1960	H=0.9 F=0.7	Norway
Lommatzsch et al. 1985	1976-1980	H=0.96 F=0.84	Germany
Abrahamsson, 1983	1956-1975	0.72	Sweden, west coas
Scotto et al. 1976	1969-1971	0.6	Third National Cancer Survey, United States
Mahoney et al. 1990	1975-1986	H=0.49 F=0.37	New York, United States
Dal Ri et al. 1988	1975-1984	0.54	Italy
Vidal et al. 1995	1992	0.73	France-survey national

Table I: incidence of uveal melanoma in various populations, number of cases per 100,000 inhabitants per year [3].

2.3. – Risk factors :

2.3.1. – Demographic risk factors: Essentially age, gender and socio-economic factors.

– **Age and gender :**

Uveal melanomas are exceptional before puberty, and their incidence increases with age. Singh et al [7] found 63 cases of melanoma in subjects under 20 years of age, out of a group of 8,000 cases. In almost half of these cases, the melanoma developed in the anterior uvea, but the cause of this preferential development in children remains unknown. Uveal melanoma in children therefore remains rare, and congenital uveal melanoma even more so [8,9]. In a study of uveal melanoma in children and adolescents, the age at presentation was 0 to 5 years in 3%, 5.1 to 10 years in 11%, 10.1 to 15 years in 35% and 15.1 to ≤20 in

50% [10] (Fig.1)

Table 1. Uveal melanoma in 122 children: Age at presentation by year.

Age (years)	Number (%)
0–1	0 (0)
1.1–2	0 (0)
2.1–3	1 (1)
3.1–4	1 (1)
4.1–5	2 (2)
5.1–6	3 (2)
6.1–7	0 (0)
7.1–8	4 (3)
8.1–9	2 (2)
9.1–10	5 (4)
10.1–11	1 (1)
11.1–12	5 (4)
12.1–13	17 (14)
13.1–14	9 (7)
14.1–15	11 (9)
15.1–16	10 (8)
16.1–17	9 (7)
17.1–18	6 (5)
18.1–19	13 (11)
19.1–20	23 (19)
Total	122 (100)

Fig.1: Uveal melanoma in 122 children Uveal melanoma in children and teenagers. **Saudi J Ophthalmol 2013**

The incidence of uveal melanoma increases after the fourth decade, and the mean age of patients developing uveal melanoma has progressively increased over the last 50 years, with the median age at diagnosis of uveal melanoma ranging from 59 to 62 years [11,12,13] In a recent study of epidemiological trends in uveal melanoma in 7043 patients from the SEER database (The Surveillance, Epidemiology, and End Results database) from 1973 to 2009, the mean age at diagnosis increased between 1973 (59 years) and 2009 (62 years) [13] It has been hypothesized that this upward trend is linked to increasing life expectancy and frequent eye examinations [13] However, studies from Asian countries indicate a lower age at diagnosis, with a mean age of 45 years in Chinese populations, 46 years in Asian Indians, 51 years in Taiwanese,
55 years in Japanese populations[14,15] Similarly, younger age at presentation has been reported in Hispanics at 52 years and in blacks at 54 years[16,17].

The distribution of uveal melanomas by sex shows a slight male predominance, averaging around 5% [18]. This predominance could be due to increased exposure to certain risk factors, or to hormonal factors.

– **Breed:**
Uveal melanomas mainly affect the Caucasian race; in highly pigmented individuals, the incidence is low. Analysis of the literature shows that melanodermal patients are less affected than the Caucasian race, with only 10 patients of African race among 3586 cases treated for melanoma at *Wills Eye Hospital* in Philadelphia between 1974 and 1989, and only 8 of the 1527 patients enucleated for melanoma in the COMS study between 1996 and 1998(0.5%) were African-Americans, these estimates may underestimate the true incidence of uveal melanoma in melanodermal individuals, in view of the difficulty of access to care for the African-American population [19] Data from the African continent show a lower incidence of uveal melanoma in the native population, 1 case of melanoma among 164 ocular and orbital tumors treated between 1962

and 1992 at the Congo-Kinshasa ophthalmology clinic [20], in South Africa, Miller et al. found 1 case of melanoma in a native patient compared with 153 cases in the Caucasian population during the same observation period (1954-1978), with an estimated ratio of 1:80 [21], Malik and Sheikh in Sudan found 6 cases of uveal melanoma among 854 tumours of the eye and adnexa in the Arab part of the population [22].
The incidence of uveal melanoma is low in patients with intermediate pigmentation: Asians, North Africans, Latin Americans and Indo-Americans. In China, at the ophthalmology clinic of the first medical college in Shanghai, 65 cases of melanoma were treated between 1956 and 1975,
[23] Incidence is also low in the Middle East, such as Iran, Afghanistan and India.

There is a notable difference between the incidence of melanoma in Jews of European or American origin (0.75 per 100,000 inhabitants), Jews of African origin (0.21-0.23 cases per 100,000 inhabitants), Jews of Asian origin (0.16-0.28 cases per 100,000 inhabitants) and non-Jews (0.13-0.16 cases per 100,000 inhabitants), a difference which may be linked essentially to the degree dskin pigmentation within the same population group. Jews born in Israel had lower rates than those born in Europe and America in the 1960s, but in the 1980s the situation was reversed. The results suggest that differences in rates between population groups and over time result from constitutional factors or the direct or indirect effect of solar radiation, whether early in life or from cumulative exposure [3]. Melanoma is also rare in Lebanon [24] and Morocco.

Data in the literature on the incidence of uveal melanoma in different ethnic groups and races show that the incidence is inversely proportional to the degree of skin pigmentation. They also suggest that melanoma develops at a younger age in melanodermal people than in the white population; these findings need to be verified, and are thought to be due to a difference in life expectancy, and probably to individual genetic factors [3].

Harbour et al , in a series of 65 cases of uveal melanoma, found an unexpected association between dark choroidal pigmentation and posterior uveal melanoma in white patients with clear irises, indeed increased choroidal pigmentation, due to an increase in the density of pigmented choroidal melanocytes, is not protective but may in fact be a risk factor for the development of posterior uveal melanoma in white patients[25].

–   **Socioeconomic factors**: no significant role.

2.3.2. – **Constitutional risk factors:** essentially malignant transformation of choroideal nevi, the role of ocular and oculo-palpebral melanocytosis, pregnancy, heredity and the role of iris color.

–   **Nevi** : nevi may be at the origin of certain iris melanomas, but their role in the genesis of uveal melanomas remains controversial. It is difficult to provide documented proof of the de novo genesis of a melanoma, or to demonstrate the pre-existence of a nevus in the site of a melanoma.1), or alterations in the EP (photo.2) that would have previously covered a nevus [3].

The annual rate of malignant transformation of a choroidal nevus was estimated at 1 in 8845 in the American white population [26].

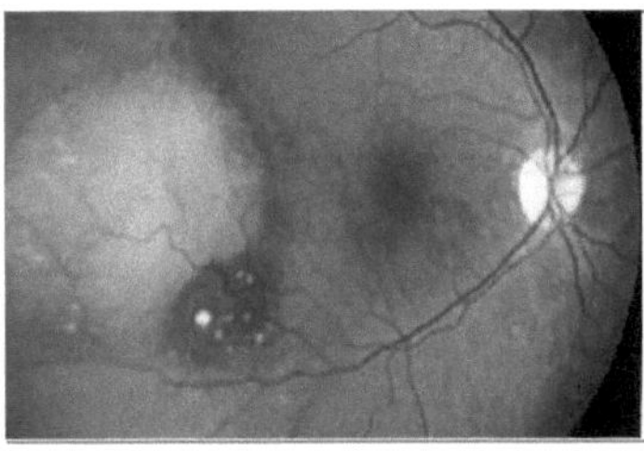 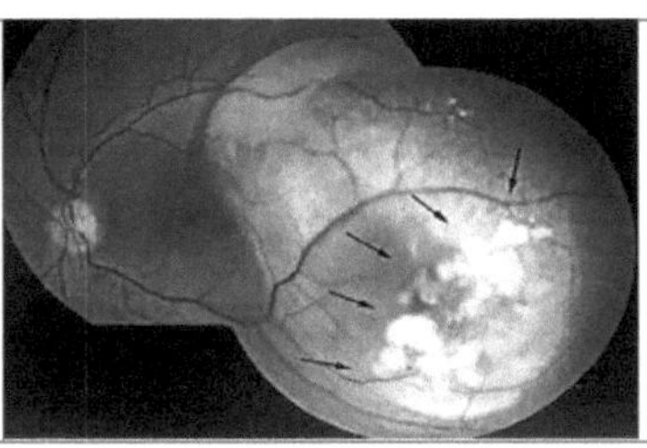

Photo.1: achromic melanoma in contact with a druse-covered nevus [Tumeurs intraoculaires rapport SFO].

photo.2: Choroidal melanoma composed of a distal island of coalescing druse (arrows) suggesting the existence of a nevus at this site **[Tumeurs intraoculaires rapport SFO]**.

–   **Ocular and oculo-palpebral melanocytosis:** elements
Melanocytosis corresponds clinically to an increase in melanocytes in all ocular tunics (photo 3) [3]. Ocular melanocytosis is more common than papular melanocytosis in Caucasians, the former more often than the latter.

The second is associated with choroideal melanoma (9 cases out of 77 vs. 1 case out of 19), according to Jules François [benign congenital melanosis of the eye]; Gonder et al, estimated that people with ocular melanocytosis had a 35-fold higher risk of developing uveal melanoma than the rest of the population; melanomas arising from sectorial melanocytosis always originate in the hyperpigmented part of the globe, and the histological structure of these melanomas presents no particularities [27]. One exception is described by Blodi [28], who reports the occurrence of a melanoma in a person with a melanocytosis, and a case of palpebral melanocytosis with uveal melanoma without ocular melanocytosis in the homolateral eye [Reichert et al. melanoma developed on OTA nevus without ocular melanosis JFO 1996] [3].

Annual fundus monitoring is recommended for people with ocular and oculo-palpebral melanocytosis, especially those in age groups at risk of developing uveal melanoma.

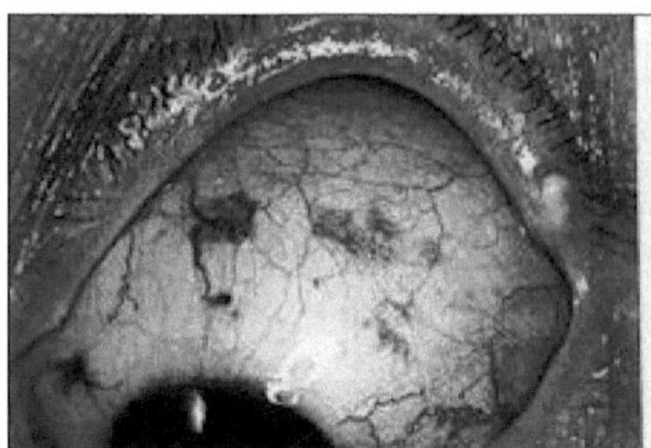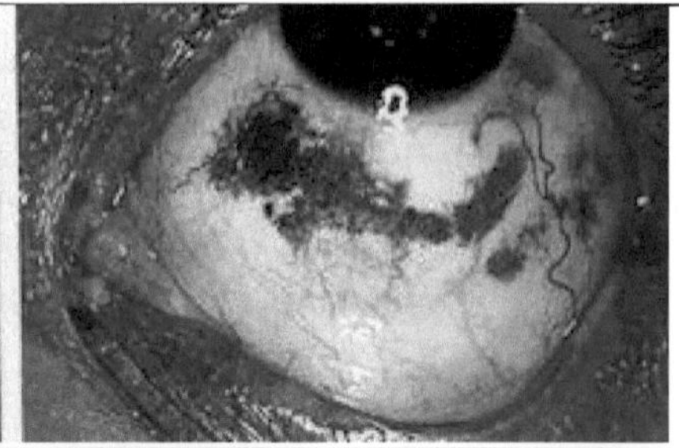

Photo 3: Ocular melanocytosis [3].

— **Hormonal factors and the role of pregnancy**: Shields et al [29] reported 16 cases of uveal melanoma diagnosed in pregnant women, with no significant differences in histopathology or survival compared to the non-pregnant group.

Tests for estrogen and progesterone receptors in ocular and metastatic melanomas, carried out by various groups, have proved negative, implying that uveal melanomas do not respond to estrogenic hormonal stimulation. [Seddon et al., 30]

Another hormonal mechanism that may be involved in the incidence and evolution of uveal melanoma is that of MSH (Melanocytic Stimulating Hormone), whose levels increase during pregnancy. However, its role in the oncogenesis of cutaneous and uveal melanomas is still poorly elucidated; this hormone, which has a regulatory effect on normal uveal melanocytes, no longer seems to retain this effect on cells transformed into melanoma. [31]

— **Hereditary factors :**

There is strong evidence that hereditary factors play a role in the development of uveal melanoma. Familial forms of uveal melanoma are extremely rare (around 1% of uveal melanomas, i.e. around 5 familial cases in France per year). Until now, the only known predisposition for uveal melanoma was an inherited alteration in the *BAP1* gene - a tumour suppressor gene - which accounts for a proportion of familial cases of uveal melanoma. [**33**]

BAP1 (BRCA1-associated protein 1) is a nuclear protein encoded by the tumor suppressor gene located on chromosome 3p21.1. BAP1 tumor predisposition syndrome is a recently identified hereditary cancer syndrome. Somatic or germline mutation of BAP1 predisposes patients to develop uveal melanoma, malignant mesothelioma, cutaneous melanomas,basal cell carcinoma and renal cell carcinoma. [34] This mutation is inherited in a Mendelian fashion, with 50% of offspring inheriting the mutation. Malignant tumors arising in patients with germline BAP1 mutations are less aggressive compared to patients with the same tumor types who do not have this mutation. An examination of 507 blood samples from uveal melanoma patients revealed 25 (5%) BAP1 polymorphisms and are associated with larger tumors and higher rates of ciliary body involvement.

The Institut Curie team has recently reported a number of cases associated with significant tumor mutation rates linked to *MBD4* gene inactivation, and which could benefit from immunotherapy. The *MBD4* (*Methyl-CpG Binding Domain 4, DNA Glycosylase*) gene codes for an enzyme involved in DNA repair and appears to act as a tumor suppressor gene. Its inactivation leads to the accumulation of a very specific type of mutation, the same that occurs as an individual or cell ages. This study analyzed over 1,000 cases of uveal melanoma patients diagnosed at the Institut Curie. For each of them, they systematically looked for the presence or absence of *MBD4* mutations in blood cells, i.e. in the patient's hereditary heritage. They identified 8 deleterious *MBD4* mutations and showed that inactivation of this gene was associated with a high rate of mutations in the tumors of these patients, demonstrating that this is a new predisposition gene for uveal melanoma.
Germline mutations of *MBD4* give a relative risk: an individual carrying
10 times more likely to develop uveal melanoma.

than a person without the mutation. *That said, uveal melanoma is a very rare disease. Although the risk of developing it is 10 times greater, it remains a rare probability in an individual's lifetime* [**33**].

In MBD4 metastatic uveal melanoma, monosomy 3 is associated with a shorter metastasis-free interval compared with disomy 3 rather than a higher relapse rate. [35]

− **Iris color, skin tone and tanning ability:**
Ten studies (1732 cases) provided information on the association between light (blue and grey) versus dark (brown) irises and the occurrence of uveal melanoma. In this meta-analysis, light irises were shown to be associated with a 75% increased risk of developing uveal melanoma, **There are** two likely explanations for this association: firstly, eyes with lighter irises generally have less melanin in the choroid and retinal pigment epithelium, and are therefore less protected against UV light. Secondly, lighter irises may be a predisposing phenotype unrelated to the amount of melanin. Unfortunately, this study was unable to distinguish between these 2 hypotheses. [36]

Based on data from five studies (586 cases), light skin color was a statistically significant risk factor for the development of uveal melanoma. [36]

Six studies (1021 cases) provided information on the association of patient tanning ability and the risk of developing uveal melanoma. Thus, tanning ability was a statistically significant risk f a c t o r   f o r   the development of uveal melanoma. [36] Clearly, uveal melanoma is more common in people who sunburn easily than in those who tan well.

The preferential location of iris melanomas in the lower half of the iris, which is more exposed to UV rays, is an argument in favor of the role played by environmental factors [3].

2.3.3. – Exogenous risk factors :

–   **Sun exposure :**

Various studies have explored the specific association between exposure to ultraviolet radiation and the occurrence of uveal melanoma. [37,38] However, the published literature does not unequivocally implicate sun exposure as a risk factor for uveal melanoma. [37,38] Shah *et al*, provided a meta-analysis of all published reports and demonstrated that chronic exposure to ultraviolet radiation, occupational exposure to the sun, exposure to outdoor recreation in the sun and geographical latitude of birth played a minimally significant role in the development of uveal melanoma [37]. A study in Germany found that people with clear irises had an increased risk of melanoma if exposed to ultraviolet radiation. [38] The Odds Ratio (OR) was 3.0 in certain at-risk professions, notably ship captains, fishermen and sailors, who were subjected to intense UV exposedebreverberation from the surface of the water; there was no increase in the OR for agricultural occupations. [39]

–   **Intermittent exposure to artificial UV :**

Some studies suggest that occupational exposure to artificial UV is a significant risk factor for the development of uveal melanoma in arc welders, OR 8.3 [39], [40]. Increasing evidence suggests that exposure to blue light, relative to UV exposure, may influence the oncogenesis and progression of uveal melanoma. [41] In a meta-analysis of five case-control studies, it was suggested that professional cooking was associated with an increased risk of uveal melanoma in men and women [42].

•**Exposure to certain chemicals:** Industrial exposure to oncogenic chemicals may play a role in the pathogenesis of uveal melanoma. For example, several cases of ocular cancer were reported among employees of the Dupont-Belle West Virginia chemical plant between 1952 and 1978. However, the epidemiologists responsible for this investigation were unable to determine the cause of these numerous cases [43].

Chapter III:
Clinical presentation of melanoma of the choroid and ciliary body :

According to various statistical estimates, 80-90% of ocular melanomas occur in the posterior uvea [44].

3.1– Symptomatology: non-specific but can sometimes be suggestive, the most frequent complaint is decreased visual acuity (48.8%), when the tumor is choroidal, this decrease in acuity results from extension of the RSD into the macular region, disorders of the media, or tumor invasion of the macula[3].
When the tumor is located in the ciliary body, visual impairment is associated wth crystalline astigmatism or sectorial opacities in the lens [3].
When visual impairment is discreet, it is often described as a "veil" [3].
Around 10 to 30% of patients report photopsia, scotomas, myodesopsia, metamorphopsia or micropsia; around 1 to 9% of patients report xanthopsia, pain, ocular inflammation, tearing, oscillopsia or loss of stereoscopic vision; the presence ddilated episcleral vessels is reported by 9.2% of sufferers (Photo 4), while an episcleral tumour nodule rarely alerts the patient (1.2%) (Photo 4.c) [3]. Less than 1% of patients complain of monocular diplopia, visual fatigue, reduced sensitivity to light, loss of color vision, photophobia, hyperopia or night blindness [44].
Around 10% of cases are asymptomatic, generally corresponding to small or medium-sized tumors located near the equator, discovered accidentally during a routine fundus examination [44].
Annular melanoma of the ciliary body, a rare entity (0.3%) of all uveal melanomas, the tumor extends circumferentially to the entire ciliary body, often without a nodular component [45].

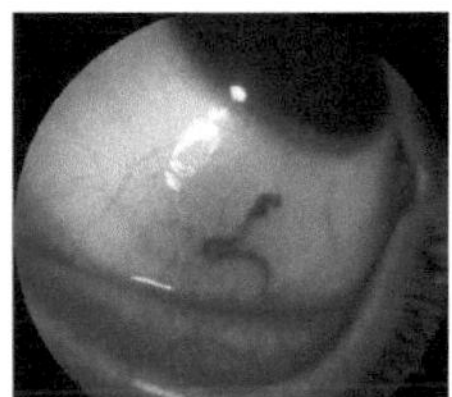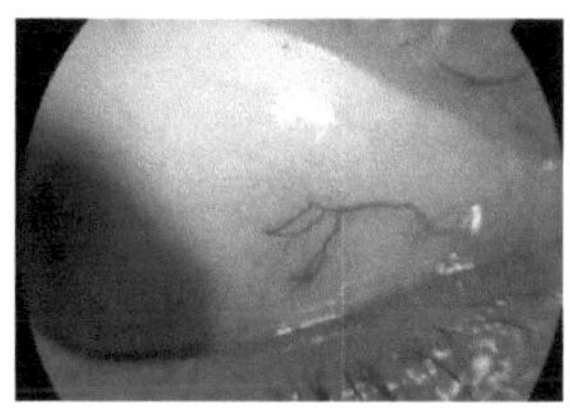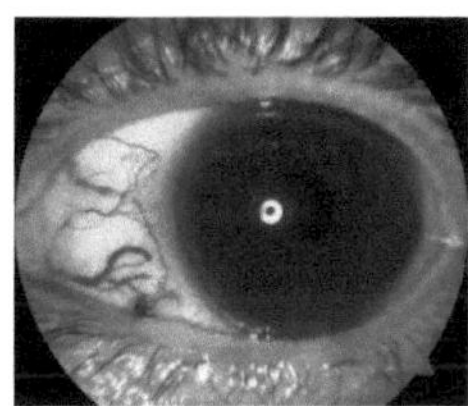

Photo 4: AS photos: (a) dilated episcleral vessel in the setting of a ciliary body melanoma, (b) dilated episcleral vessel in the setting of a choroideal melanoma, (c) dilated episcleral vessels, with episcleral tumor nodule in relation to a choroidal melanoma EHS ophthalmology Oran, Mesri.Kh

3.2. – Melanoma of the choroid :

3.2.1. – Melanoma pigmentation: melanoma is usually grey or greenish-brown, but can vary in color from dark brown to creamy white. Tumor pigmentation is sometimes heterogeneous. Melanoma must be distinguished from solitary metastases [44].

3.2.2. – Size and shape: axial tumor growth is contained by the sclera, so that the tumor protrudes into the vitreous cavity; small and medium-sized tumors that are still contained by an intact Bruch's membrane are dome-shaped (fig. 2 a); if Bruch's membrane ruptures at the apex of the tumor, the melanoma will be mushroom-shaped (fig. 2 b), if it ruptures at the edge of the tumor, the latter develops an irregular, sloping shape [44] by rupturing Bruch's membrane, melanoma can invade the retina and vitreous cavity giving a particular entity is rare (0.4%) of choroidal melanomas, Knapp-Ronne melanoma, which is characterized by its location close to the papilla, its early penetration of the sensory retina with vitreous invasion, its histology is characterized by blood-filled, bloodless cavernous spaces and its frequent manifestation is massive vitreous hemorrhage [46].

In a review of 7256 cases of choroidal melanoma, the mean basal diameter was 11.3mm and the mean thickness was 5.2mm [11]

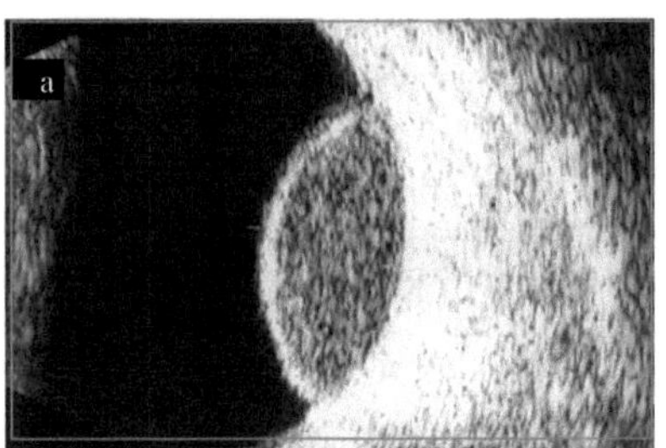
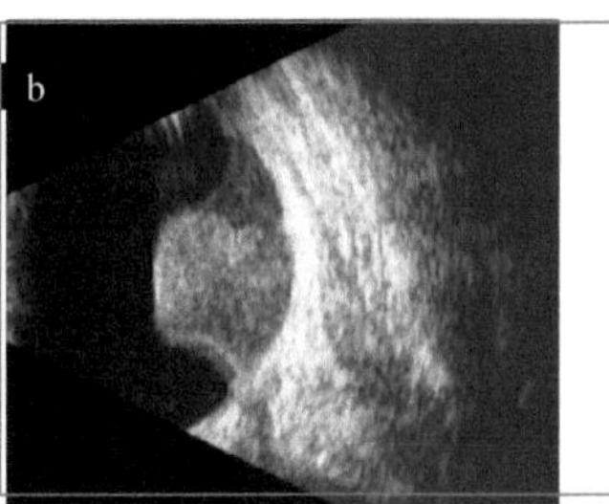

Fig. 2: (a) Ultrasonographically dome-shaped melanoma, 6 mm thick,
(b) mushroom-shaped melanoma on ultrasonography, (b) **[44]**

Diffuse melanoma is a special, infiltrative, flat or slightly elevated entity with predominantly horizontal growth, defined by Reese and Howard [48] as a tumor whose surface area exceeds ¼ of the choroidal surface, and whose thickness does not exceed 5 mm, with an irregular surface, heterogeneous pigmentation, and a tendency to extend extra-sclerally, or glaucoma if it invades the anterior segment (photo5) Some melanomas have a nodular part and a diffuse part, the growth pattern having changed during development (photo5) others arise from sectorial melanocytosis, the margins of which are difficult to distinguish from the rest of the pigmentation (photo8) another variant is multi-nodular melanoma, which arises from polyclonal tumour cell lines that develop with different doubling times (photo5)[44].

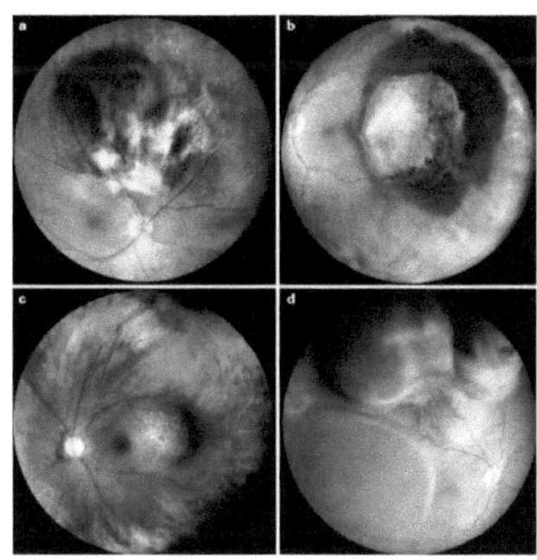

Photo 5: Growth patterns of uveal melanomas: **a**: diffuse choroidal melanoma, irregular surface, heterogeneous pigmentation, maximum thickness 3mm on B-mode ultrasonography, **b**: choroidal melanoma with a nodular and diffuse portion, **c**: temporal choroidal melanoma developing on sectorial melanocytosis, **d**: upper multi-nodular melanoma with bullous DSR [44

3.2.3. – Variants: some melanomas can be distinguished by specific growth sites, giving them typical clinical characteristics.

–   **Small melanoma of the posterior pole: a** real diagnostic challenge, to be differentiated from choroidal nevus (photo6) the main risk factors are ocular symptomatology, retinal edema or sub-retinal fluid [49] (photo6) absence of druses, presence of self-fluorescing orange pigments [50] (photo6), the presence of pinpoints on fluorescein angiography (photo9) and a thickness of more than 2 mm on ultrasound or EDI-OCT [51] the diagnosis of melanoma is generally made clinically on the basis of documented growth during periodic surveillance [51].

–   **Small peripapillary melanoma:** when Bruch's membrane is intact, a tumor at this site can sometimes encircle the optic disc. The increased thickness of the tumor may cause Bruch's membrane to rupture at the edge of the disc, resulting in a tumor nodule covering the disc. This type of tumor is similar in appearance to papillary melanocytoma [44].

•**Multifocal and bilateral melanomas:** are rare and have been reported in a limited number of cases [3].

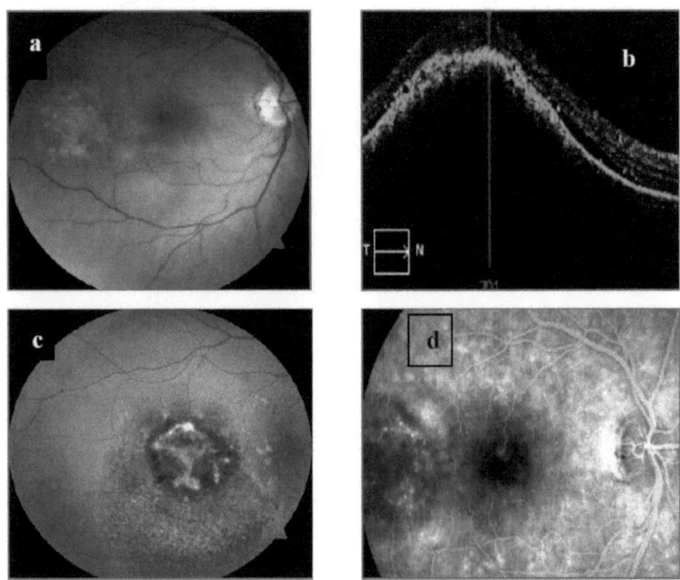

Photo6: (a) small posterior pole melanoma in a 57-year-old Caucasian man, (b) DSR, (c) self-fluorescent orange pigments, (d) angio-fluo pinpoints. EHS ophthalmology Oran, Mesri.Kh

3.2.4. – Décol

3.2.5. Retinal detachment: Choroidal melanoma is almost always accompanied by exudative retinal detachment. The presence of sub-retinal fluid can be detected as early as possible with OCT [50]. It spreads progressively from the tumor surface to the lower periphery and macular region. The retinal surface is usually smooth, and the sub-retinal fluid may be clear or cloudy [44].

The more extensive and chronic the retinal detachment, the greater the risk of ischemia and telangiectasia, factors which must be taken into account during treatment and follow-up.

In some cases, pigmented cells accumulate in the sub-retinal fluid, demarcating the edges of the retinal detachment. These cells are mainly pigment-laden macrophages, sometimes mixed with tumor cells. The melanoma associated with this type of complication often has an epithelioid or necrotic histological appearance, with poor cell cohesion. Disseminated pigmented cells may also be seen in the vitreous cavity when the retina is invaded, or when the tumor is located in the ciliary body [44].

3.2.6. – Intraocular pressure: Around 3% of uveal melanomas are associated with secondary glaucoma at the time of diagnosis [82]. The mechanisms generally responsible for elevated intraocular pressure are tumour invasion of the iridocorneal angle and neovascularization of the iris. Rarely, glaucoma is secondary to anterior displacement of the iridocrystalline block, due to the large volume and anterior location of the tumour.

Melanomas invading the ciliary body may induce a relative decrease in intraocular pressure, probably due to disruption of ciliary epithelial function [44].

3.2.7. – Inflammatory reaction: very large melanomas are often accompanied by a moderate inflammatory reaction, the severity of which correlates with the thickness of the tumour, the extent of exudative retinal detachment and the presence of necrosis, leukocyte infiltration and haemorrhage [53,54]. In some cases, the inflammatory reaction may lead to synechiae, resulting in pupillary block. Exceptionally, the inflammatory reaction may take the form of scleritis or episcleritis [55], endophthalmitis [56] or orbital cellulitis [57].

3.2.8. – Extra-scleral extension :

T h e sclera offers considerable resistance to the expansion of these tumors, but it is crossed by channels that can be used by tumor cells, Melanomas of the ciliary body externalize through the aqueous veins and anterior ciliary arteries, while melanomas of the posterior uvea externalize through the scleral canals of the vorticose veins and posterior ciliary arteries. Externalizing nodules may rupture as they increase in volume, invading the orbit (photo 7); flat melanomas, large tumours composed of epithelioid cells, highly pigmented tumours, melanomas infiltrating Bruch's lamina, are the most frequently externalizing tumours [58].

A case of extra-scleral extension of a uveal melanoma after phacoemulsification has been described by our team (photo 7), a presentation never described before. However, like any externalization, it constitutes a poor prognostic factor favoring both the risk of metastasis and orbital recurrence [58].

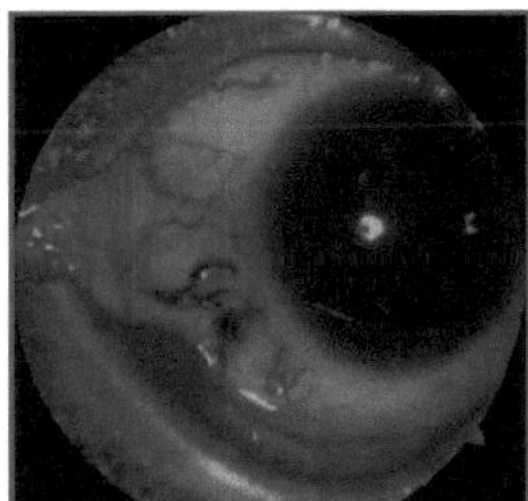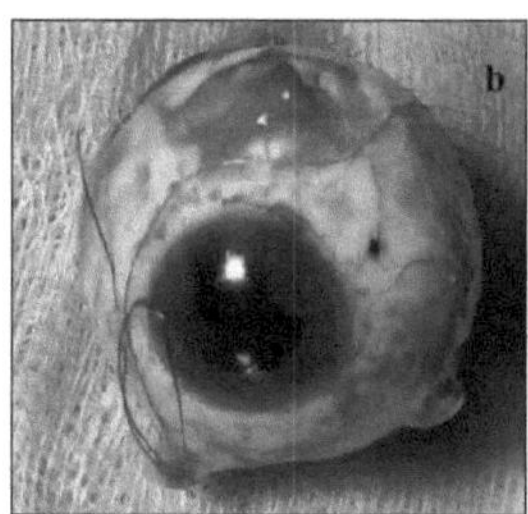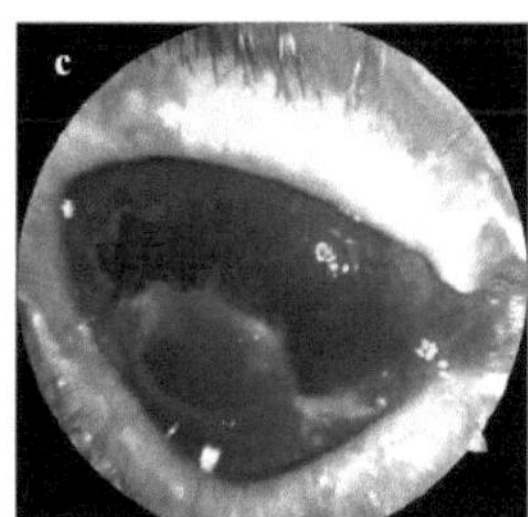

Photo 7: (a) externalizing nodule, (b) macroscopic image of an episcleral externalizing nodule, (c) massive extra-scleral externalization of a uveal melanoma after Phacoemulsification.
EHS ophthalmology Oran Mesri.Kh

3.2.9. – Optic nerve invasion: Tumor invasion of the optic disc and optic nerve is rare. It is usually secondary to a large peripapillary tumor and often associated with elevated intraocular pressure and the epithelioid or necrotic form of melanoma. However, ciliary body tumours can also lead to invasion of the optic disc and optic nerve, due to the dissemination of tumour cells into the vitreous cavity. This type of retino-invasive extension, described by Kivelä and Summanen [59], has been reported in a limited number of cases. Invasion of the optic nerve is generally limited to the part of the nerve close to the posterior scleral wall [44]. The absence of light perception and an afferent pupillary defect should raise suspicion of optic nerve invasion by a tumor located in contact with the optic disc (Fig. 3) [44].

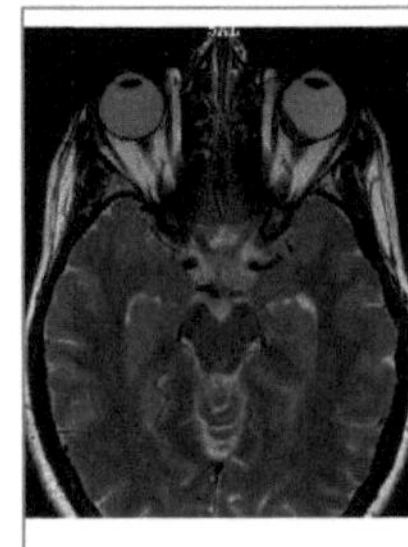

Fig. 3: Invasion of the optic nerve by a peripapillary tumor,
EHS ophthalmology Oran

3.3.   – Melanoma of the ciliary body :
Melanoma of the ciliary body may be circumscribed or annular. Slit-lamp examination, gonioscopy, transillumination and 20-50 MHz ultrasound are used to detect it and guide therapeutic management [3].

3.3.1. – Circumscribed melanoma of the ciliary body: nodular in shape and, at the time of diagnosis, generally larger than melanoma of the iris. In its early stages, this tumor is confined to the ciliary body and is therefore asymptomatic. Ciliary body melanoma is usually brown, corresponding to the color of the overlying pigment epithelium, unless the latter has been invaded by the tumor, in which case the true color of the tumor becomes visible. On 20-50 MHz US, its structure may be homogeneous or heterogeneous and sometimes associated with cysts [44]

3.3.1.1.   – Growth: Melanomas of the ciliary body generally displace rather than infiltrate the iris root and invade the anterior chamber (photo 11), where they become visible on gonioscopy. They can seed

cells throughout the anterior chamber, on the iris surface and in the iridocorneal angle, leading to pressure elevation. Melanomas can also spread around the ciliary body in an annular fashion, and this pattern of growth should be ruled out in all cases at 20-50 MHz US [44]

3.3.1.2. – **Complications**: In addition to glaucoma, as melanoma of the ciliary body thickens, it progressively compresses the equator of the lens, causing sectorial opacities and consequent loss of visual acuity (photo 8). In more advanced stages, lens deformation will occur in younger patients, while in older patients with a thickened lens
"more rigid", subluxation or dislocation of the lens is more likely [44].

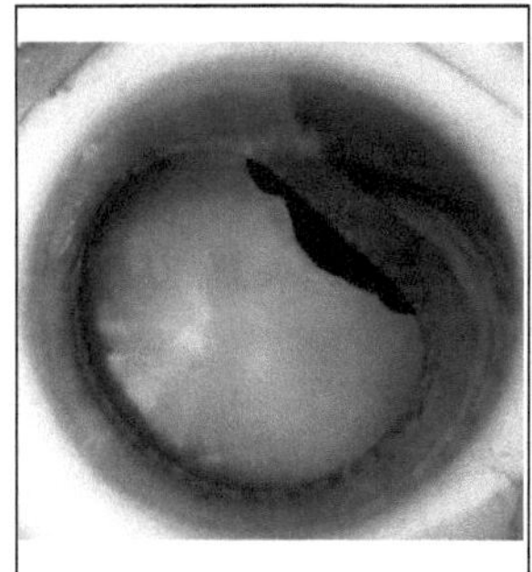

Photo 8: Melanoma of the ciliary body displacing and infiltrating the iris root, invading the anterior chamber and causing secondary cataract [74].

3.3.2. – **Circumferential melanoma of the ciliary body**: the diagnosis is usually made after it has grown considerably. There is usually more than 180° of ciliary body circumference involved, and disproportionately less anteroposterior growth. Occasionally, it may develop as a secondary extension of an anterior choroidal melanoma [44]. The presence of sentinel vessels, sectorial cataract, unilateral glaucoma and unexplained iridocyclitis should raise suspicion of circumferential ciliary body melanoma [45]. Detailed evaluation with slit-lamp examination, gonioscopy, transillumination and 20-50 MHz ultrasound is necessary to establish the diagnosis and guide the most appropriate treatment.

Anamnesis: personal and family, all the information gathered is taken into account in the diagnostic approach and choice of treatment [3].

4.1. – **Ocular examination:** initially includes examination of the contralateral eye, which is important because certain pathologies and pseudotumors can mimic uveal melanoma. In some cases, the condition of the contralateral eye determines the radical or conservative attitude of the affected eye, and bilateral melanoma is very rare but possible [3].

The ophthalmological examination includes measurement of corrected and uncorrected VA, complete biomicroscopy, tonometry, gonioscopy, and examination of the FO [3] Ophthalmoscopy   indirect   binocular   with   lateral indentations   allows observation of the tumor and exudative retinal detachment in relief, complemented by a detailed drawing of the FO (Fig.4), Damato.B has proposed a mnemonic method MELANOMA to alert the practitioner to an intraocular tumor when the pupils are not dilated.

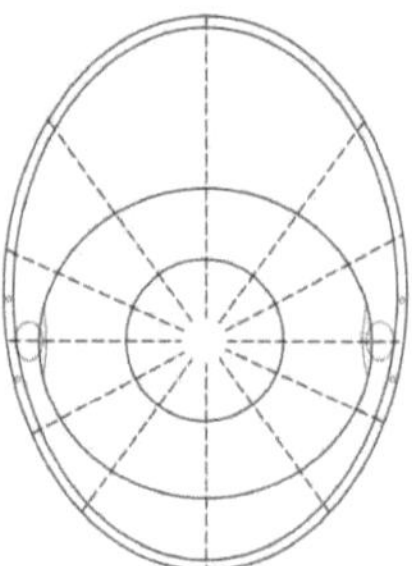

Fig.4: Template for reporting examination results using a fenestration lamp

4.2. – **General examination:** indicated in all patients with uveal melanoma, in search of metastatic dissemination, even if only 1-3% of patients have metastases at the time of diagnosis of the disease.

intraocular tumor, and that metastatic sites only become detectable after months or years of tumor treatment. A general clinical examination is recommended, as well as serum alkaline phosphatase, serum glutamo-oxaloacetic transaminase

(GOT) and serum glutamopyruvic transaminase (GPT), given the preponderance of hepatic involvement, and a thoracic-abdominal-pelvic (TAP) scan. If the results are positive, the search for metastases should be extended, and even a biopsy of the metastatic site should be performed to confirm the diagnosis [3].

4.3. – Fluorescein and indocyanine green angiography :

The angiographic appearance of choroideal melanomas depends on several parameters, including the degree of pigmentation of the tumor, its vascularization, its structure, the state of the pigmentary epithelium and the retina. Uveal melanomas present an angiographic polymorphism.

In small and medium-sized melanomas, there are surface alterations and changes in the angiostructure of the tumor, with surface alterations present in the early sequences of fluorescein angiography, alternating hyperflurescent areas corresponding to PE alterations, and hypoflurescent, shielding areas corresponding to orange pigment or petechiae; in late sequences, exudation phenomena appear on the tumor surface or peri-tumoral [3].

On the surface of melanomas, in late venous sequences, hyper-fluorescent pinpoints are frequently observed. These lesions may be on the surface or in a circle around the tumor (photo 12), and their location may change over time. Histopathologically, pinpoints may correspond to hyaline glycolipido-protein droplets, which sit in contact with Bruch's membrane.

Fluorescein angiography can also reveal a lift or a Blow-out fracture of the EP, and nodules on the tumor surface, if the retina is infiltrated; their angiographic behavior depends on their degree of pigmentation [3].

Typically, melanoma gives a double-network appearance on early images (achromic tumors) (photo 9), with inhomogeneous fluorescein impregnation on late images with pinpoints. [3]

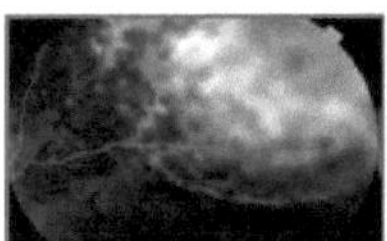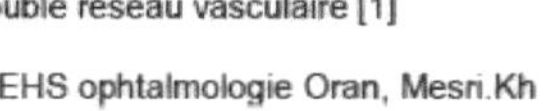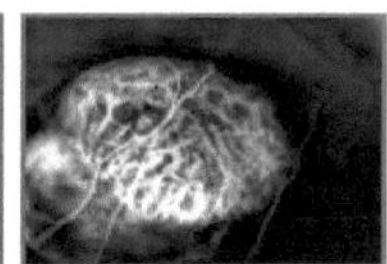

Photo 9: (a) séquences tardives d'angiographie à la fluorescéine avec pinpoints, EHS ophtalmologie Oran, Mesri.Kh   (b) volumineux mélanome de la choroide, aspect de double réseau vasculaire [1]

EHS ophtalmologie Oran, Mesri.Kh   (c) Aspect en double réseau aux temps précoces (tumeurs achromes) Shields Intraocular tumors Atlas 2015

Indocyanine green angiography enables us to study tumor and peri-tumor vascularization, tumor surface alterations, the appearance of exudation and its peri-tumoral diffusion. Intra-tumor vascularization is characterized by its tortuosity, irregularity and tendency to exudate, and its tendency to exude (photo 10); dilatation of the tumour drainage system, extending as far as the ampulla of vorticosis, is most often observed on ICG in small and medium-sized melanomas, while large tumours appear to be pushing back the large vascular trunks of the choroidea. ICG is particularly useful in cases of diagnostic doubt with hemangiomas (photo 10) [3].

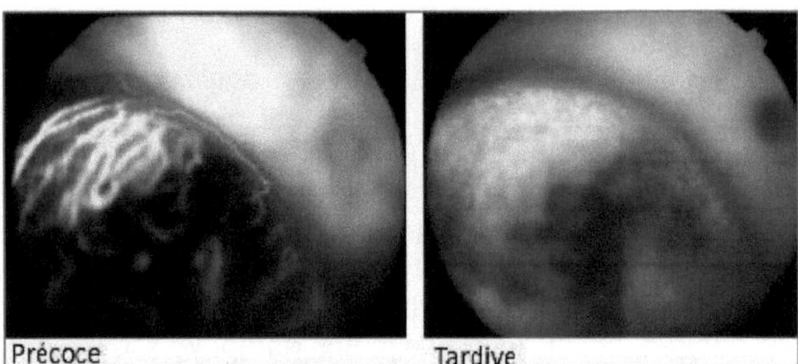

Photo 10 : Comparaison entre l'angio ICG du mélanome versus hémangiome,
a) Vascularisation tumorale bien visible (tumeurs achromes)
Précoce: surface tumorale hypocyanescente
Tardive: hypercyanescence modérée Shields Atlas 3rd Ed

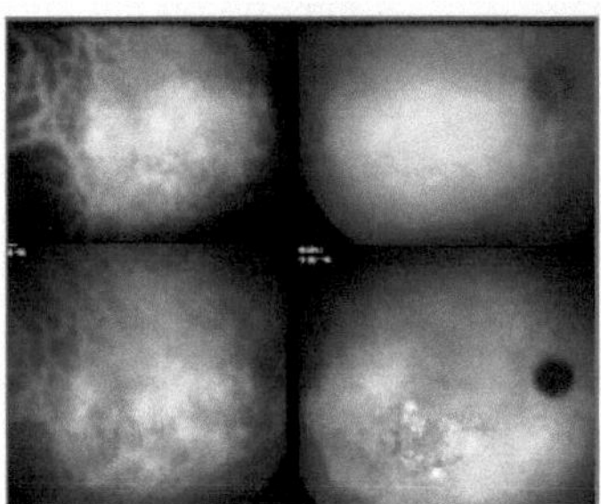

b) Remplissage précoce avec vaisseaux nourriciers visibles, accentuation de la fluorescence, décroissance tardive (Wash out), persistance possible de points fluorescents qui peuvent correspondre à la coloration de cavités tumorales [HEMANGIOME CHOROIDIEN Margaret STERKERS]

In secondary retinal detachments, indocyanine green, impregnates the LSR and marks its edges, fluorescein forms a bright, blurred corona. [3]

Gravitational epitheliopathy may accompany melanomas, it may be cicatricial or active, the former tends to give early hyperfluorescence without diffusion on fluorescein angiography, and hypocyanescence in late sequences on ICG, the latter gives late hyperfluorescence in both examinations (photo 11)[3].

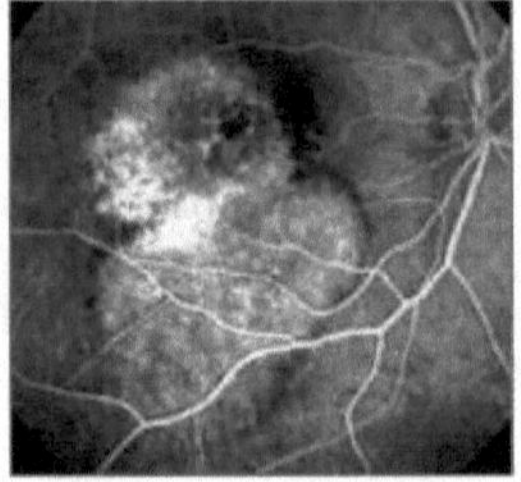

Photo 11 : Image fluoroangiographique d'une épithéliopathie gravitationnelle, plage ovalaire qui comprend des altérations de type cicatriciel de l'EP, en dessous et à cheval sur la marge tumorale **[3]**

–   4.5. – **Ultrasonography:**   ultrasonography   is   the   most   useful complementary examination for diagnosing melanomas of the choroidea and ciliary body, particularly in the case of media disorders. It enables us to study the shape, measurements and echo structure of the tumour, and to assess the integrity of the scleral wall. Transvitreal A and B ultrasonography techniques are used for melanomas of the posterior uvea, and high-frequency or medium-frequency immersion B ultrasonography for melanomas of the ciliary body [3].

–   **Ultrasonography A**: useful for tumors over 2-3 mm thick.
Choroidal melanoma characteristically presents a prominent initial spike, followed by low reflectivity, ranging from 10% to 60% of the scleral peak. Melanoma attenuation is high, with a kappa angle greater than 45° (Fig.5). Melanomas are also richly vascularized tumors, as evidenced by rapid oscillations of the spaces between two peaks in A-mode (in 80% of cases) and the

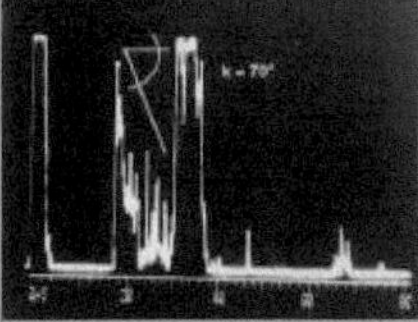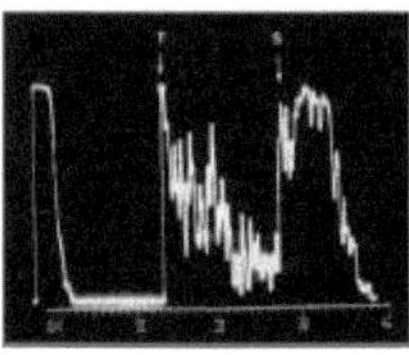

Fig. 5 : Mesure de l'angle kappa en écho A d'un mélanome de la choroide.
T : écho d'entrée tumorale. S : écho bifide de la sclérotique. T-S : volume tumoral avec réflectivité moyenne et irrégulière [3]

presence of vessels in color Doppler ultrasound (in over 95% of cases) [60].

–   **Ultrasound B**: is used to help establish the diagnosis, to assess possible extraocular extension (Fig.6), to estimate tumor size for periodic observation [61].
For biometric measurements (tumor thickness and largest basal diameter), a cut is made along the tumor's longest meridian, to measure its longitudinal diameter and thickness, followed by a cut orthogonal to this meridian, to measure its transverse diameter. It is useful to make three concordant measurements and to give the mean of each value (with a standard deviation of less than 0.10) and the maximum value. For thickness, the thickness of the tumor itself should be measured, without taking the retina or sclera into account. This must be clearly stated in the report. For the longitudinal diameter of a peripheral tumor, it is sometimes difficult, if not impossible, to visualize the most peripheral part of the mass, even if it is voluminous, especially over 6 and 12 hours. The echostructure of uveal melanoma is homogeneous, and there are never any calcifications, the excavation of the underlying uveal tissue, which corresponds to the replacement of the normal, fairly echogenic choroid by hypoechoic tumour tissue, shading the underlying soft tissues (Fig.6)[60,61].

Ultrasound biomicroscopy (UBM) offers the following advantages:Provides excellent resolution for anterior segment anomalies, including ciliary body melanomas (Fig.7)

– Can differentiate very anterior choroidal melanomas from those of ciliary origin [61].

This examination is highly operator-dependent, and requires training to ensure that examinations are of sufficient quality for diagnosis and patient follow-up.

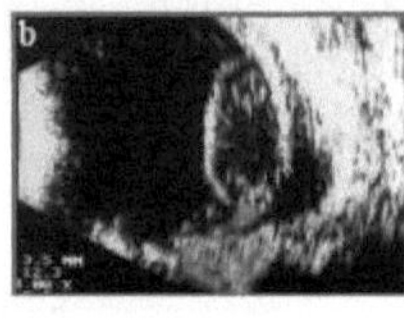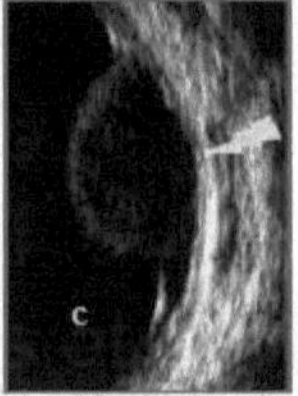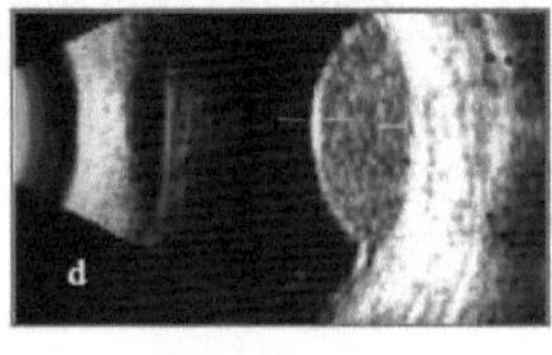

Fig.6 : b : extension extra sclérale, réflectivité moins élevée que la graisse orbitaire [3], c : mélanome de la choroide, en dôme, avec excavation choroïdienne. O. BERGES, Fondation Rothschild, d : mélanome de la choroide, en dôme, ombre portée soulignée par les pointillés violets. Extrait Clinical echography of the eye and orbit, Ad M. Verbeek.

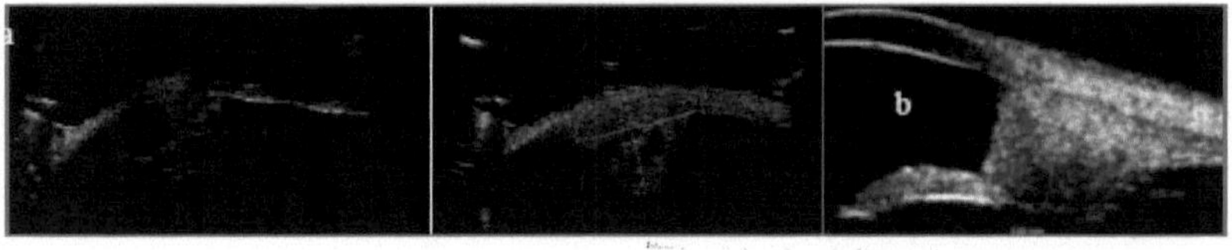

Fig. 7 : a. Tumeur du corps ciliaire avec espaces kystiques clairement définis par échographie. Images courtesy of Bertil Damato, PhD, FRCOphth, University of California, San Francisco 2013. b. aspect UBM d'un mélanome du corps ciliaire, images Alexandre Matet (institut Curie2019)|

4.4. – Optical coherence tomography (OCT) :

The diagnostic contribution of OCT in choroidal melanoma is limited to melanomas of small thickness and posterior location, and it is this type of lesion that poses the most problems of differential diagnosis. The main signs that can be studied with OCT are :

– Maximum tumor thickness,

– Bruch's membrane rupture;

– The presence of orange pigments ;

– Serous detachment of the neuroepithelium.

– Current OCTs allow only limited analysis of the mass, due to insufficient beam penetration of the choroidea, and absorption of the optical signal on the surface of the melanoma [62] (Fig.8).

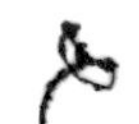

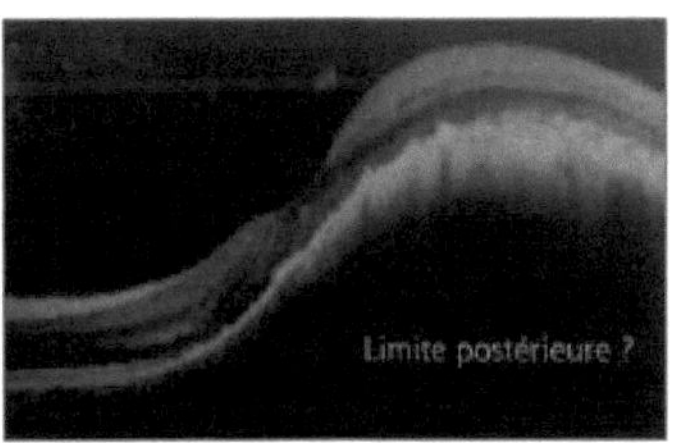

Fig.8: Coupe OCT ne permettant pas de déterminer l'épaisseur de la lésion, en raison de l'ombrage postérieur lié à la réflectivité du mélanome [62]

OCT in EDI (enhanced depth imaging spectral-domain) mode can be used to measure melanomas up to 3 mm thick with greater accuracy than ultrasound [63] (Fig.9).

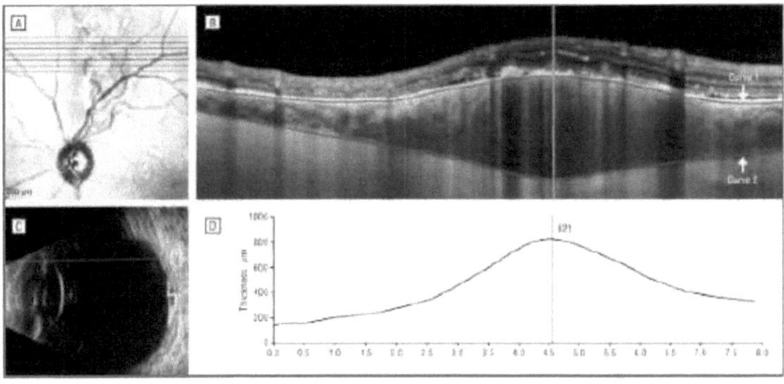

Fig.9: Évaluation d'un petit mélanome choroïdien par EDI-OCT et par échographie. A : photographie infrarouge montrant 7 vecteurs d'une image EDI-OCT passant à travers un mélanome choroïdien juxta papillaire. B : mesure l'épaisseur de la tumeur choroïdienne avec curve 1 le long du bord interne du mélanome et avec la curve 2 le long du bord externe du mélanome. C : Mesure de l'épaisseur du mélanome choroïdien de l'apex à la base de la lésion par échographie (trait jaune). D : mesure de l'épaisseur choroïdienne maximale à l'OCT entre curve1 et 2 [63].

OCT can be very useful for Bruch's membrane rupture, which is a pathognomonic sign of choroid melanomas, although rare in thin lesions. OCT enables very early

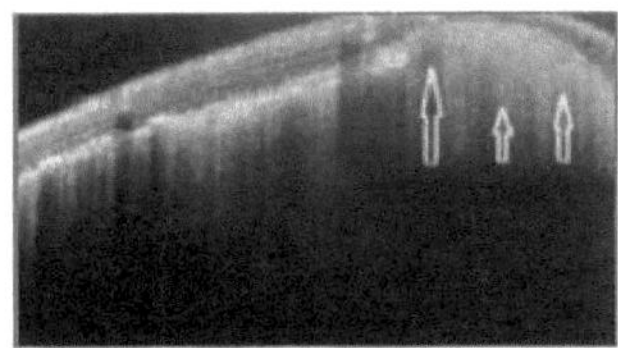

Fig. 10 : Hernie tumorale au travers de la membrane de Bruch d'une tumeur achrome [62]

diagnosis, quicker than ultrasound (Fig.10).

The presence of orange pigment on the surface of a tumor lesion is an important prognostic factor in melanoma, with Shields et al [63] emphasizing its more frequent presence in melanoma versus nevi (95% versus 45%) for Sayanagi et al. (61% versus 11%) [49] , the orange pigment is better individualized on SD-OCT than on TD-OCT, appearing as nodosities or plaques on the surface of

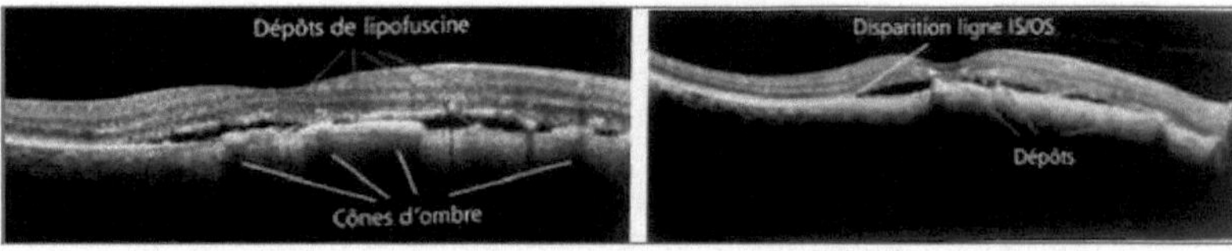

Fig.11 : mélanome plan du pôle postérieur. OCT (a, b) montre des dépôts de lipofuscine, des altérations de l'EP [62].

a | b

the EP with which it seems to be continuous; the presence of these deposits results in signal absorption, casting a shadow on the underlying choroidea, with disappearance of the ellipsoid line, on their surface, and on the surface of the tumor [49, 62] (Fig.11)

Serous detachment of the neuroepithelium (DSNE), even very discrete, aggravates the patient's metastatic risk [11], and is present more frequently in small melanomas than in nevi (92%versus16%) [63].

Shields et al [11] have described a particular morphological characteristic of photoreceptors in DSNEs, known as *shaggy photoreceptors:* hyper-reflective dots on the outer surface of the retina raised by the DSNE, overhanging certain melanomas; more or less elongated, sometimes ballooned dots (Fig.12) present in 49% of melanomas versus no cases found in nevi [63].
Histologically, *shaggy photoreceptors* correspond to macrophage proliferations adherent to the posterior surface of the retina, containing melanin granules derived from the retinal PE [64]. These lesions are thought to exist in central serous chorioretinitis, choroidal hemangiomas and metastases, but their presence in suspicious melanocytic lesions is almost pathognomonic for the diagnosis of melanoma [62].

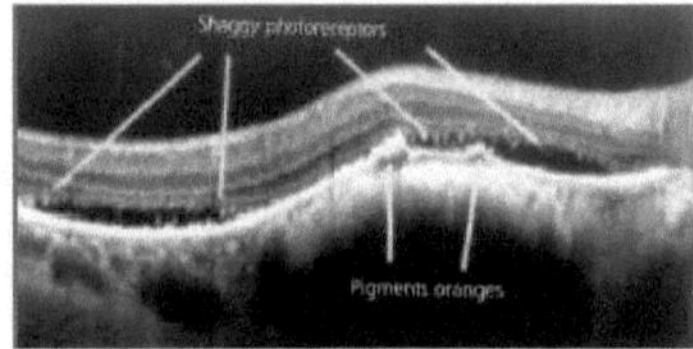

Fig.12 : liquide sous rétinien, shaggy photoreceptors, pigments orange [62]

The reflectivity of the anterior part of the choroidea, just behind the EP and in front of the choroidal melanoma, is variable and non-homogeneous depending on the patient [65], but it would seem that in melanomas, this band is hyper-reflective, thin or even absent, with a high absorption of the optical signal

[62] (Fig. 13).
The images given by OCT A are similar to those given by ICG angiography in achromic melanomas, i.e. anarchic tumor vascularization. These are surface images, due to the rapid absorption of the optical signal, and consequently this examination does not allow in-depth analysis of the tumor. [62] (Fig. 14)

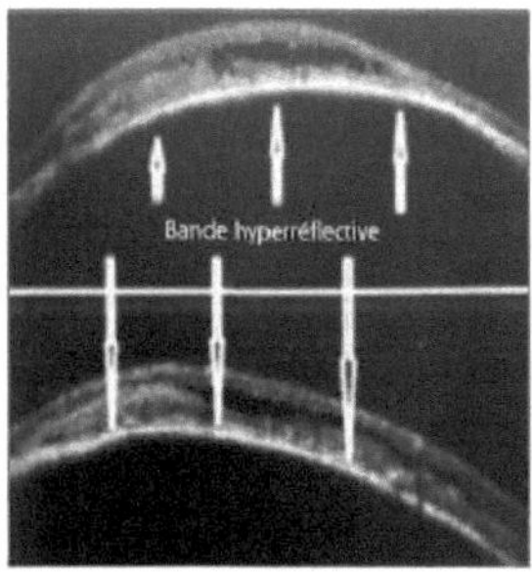
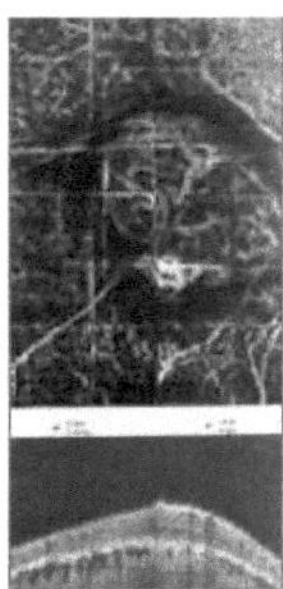

Fig.13 : mélanome avec bande hyper-réflective étroite voire absente [62]

Fig. 14 : OCT-A d'un mélanome choroïdien achrome montrant une vascularisation intra-tumorale semblable à celle mise en évidence en angio ICG [62]

The density of the vascularization of the chorio-capillary between the tumor and the EP-Bruch's membrane complex would be lower, with areas of hypodensity. It is conceivable that these changes would correspond to the hyper-reflectivity observed on OCT and described above, and could be due to the fact that the melanoma completely disorganizes this part of the chorio-capillary to the point of making it disappear **[62] (Fig. 15).**

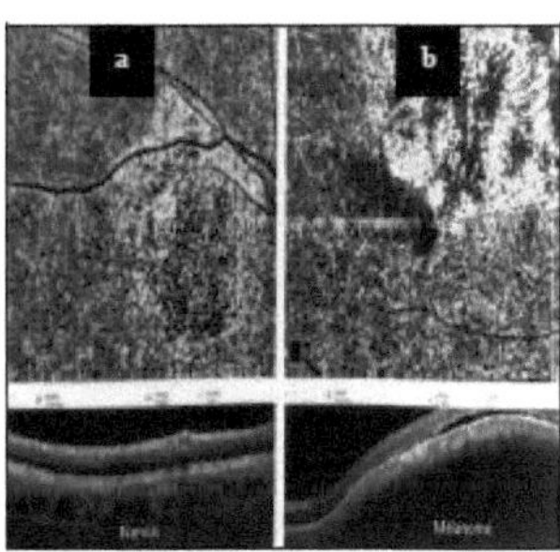
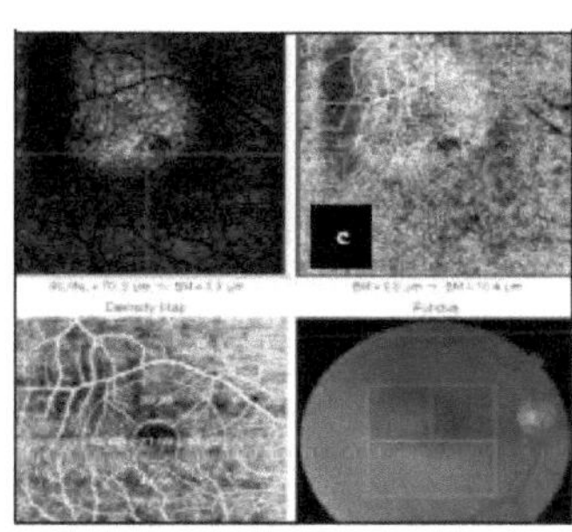

Fig. 15: la densité de la chorio-capillaire supra tumorale est normale dans un cas de nævus choroïdien (a, c) mais amoindrie, avec des espaces morts, dans un cas de mélanome choroïdien (b) **[64]**, (c) EHS Ophtalmologie d'Oran Mesri.S

4.5. – **Doppler ultrasonography:** this examination identifies and locates the large-calibre vessels present in the tumour, and estimates the speed and direction of circulation [3]. In fact, uveal melanoma is characterized by a higher maximum blood flow in the central retinal artery and posterior short ciliary arteries [66] (Figs. 16,17).

After radiotherapy, there is a decrease in blood flow and an increase in vascular resistance in the central retinal artery and posterior short ciliary arteries [66] (Fig. 18).

In addition to the qualitative superiority of EDC for assessing the vascular character of choroidal melanomas, pulsed mode provides a quantitative approach, with three stages that appear to correlate with the risk of metastasis, irrespective of the tumor's genetic profile. The absence of Doppler flow within a melanoma may be explained by massive intra-tumoral hemorrhage (e.g. thrombosis of a vorticose vein), or in the case of ocular hypertonia greater than 40 mm Hg, or at a distance from effective conservative treatment [60].

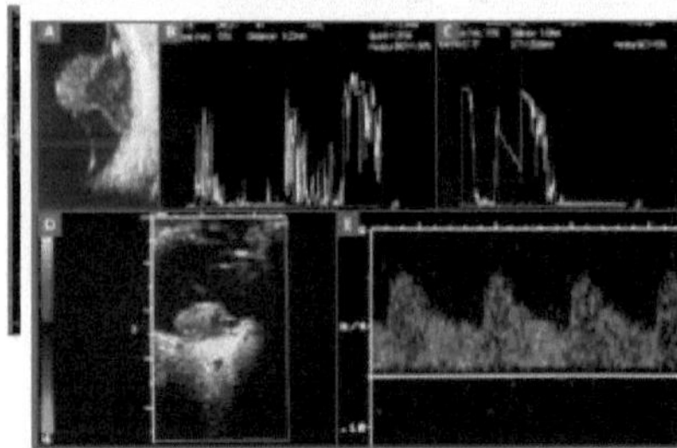

Fig. 17: Mélanome malin de la choroïde. A: Mode B, masse en bouton de col, la tête apparaissant très échogène et la base, en arrière de la lame de Bruch, hypoéchogène. L'excavation choroïdienne est nette. La lésion est entourée d'un petit décollement de rétine satellite. B: Mode A standardisé à gain standard. La réflectivité tumorale globale est faible: 38 % du pic scléral en quantification I. L'atténuation est déjà perceptible. C: Mode A standardisé avec une hauteur des pics à 50 %. L'atténuation du faisceau ultrasonore par la masse est évidente et quantifiable : angle kappa = 58°. D et E : EDC modes couleur (D) et pulsé (E). La masse parapapillaire présente une riche vascularisation arborescente artérielle, codée en rouge, provenant des artères ciliaires courtes postérieures au pôle tumoral situé près du nerf optique et des veines, codées en bleu, au pôle opposé. En mode pulsé, les flux sont rapides avec une vitesse systolique maximale de 18 cm/s [60]

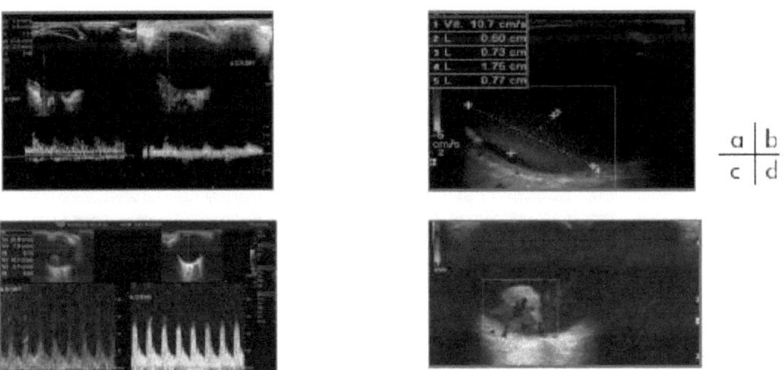

Fig.18 : a) MMC du pôle postérieur, en mode pulsé vitesse systolique maximale à 17.8 cm/s, b) mélanome malin de la choroide, avasculaire à l'Echodoppler après protonthérapie, c) en mode pulsé vitesse systolique maximale à 16.1 cm/s, d) MMC. EDC modes couleur. Mesri. Kh., Bounoua.

4.6. – MRI: Magnetic Resonance Imaging (MRI) can help diagnose melanomas in clear or opaque media, and help detect extra-scleral tumor extension or massive tumor invasion of the optic nerve [3].

MRI images of melanoma are essentially linked to the paramagnetic characteristics of melanin, i.e. a hyperintense signal compared with the vitreous in T1, hypointense in T2, with weak to moderate T1 enhancement after injection of paramagnetic contrast medium (gadolinium DTPA) (Figs. 19,20), however the diagnosis of melanoma cannot be ruled out on an atypical MRI image [3]. Current clinical MRI protocols are not optimized for MU, and T.Λ. Ferreira et al [67] have developed a device adapted for lesion characterization and assessment of local extension. Isotropic 3D Turbo-Spin Echo (TSE) sequences are more suitable for precise geometric measurements of the tumor, enabling therapeutic management planning. Diffusion-weighted and perfusion-weighted images help differentiate malignant from benign lesions and provide quantitative measurements of tumor hemodynamics and cellularity, enabling prediction and evaluation of treatment outcome.

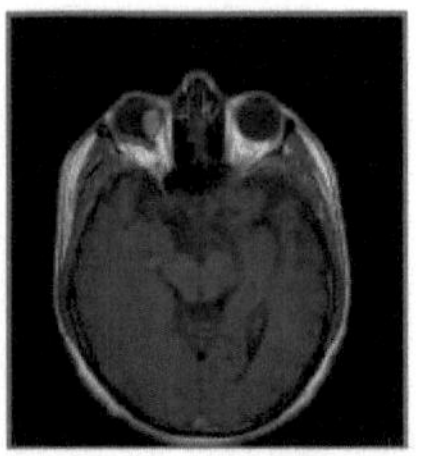 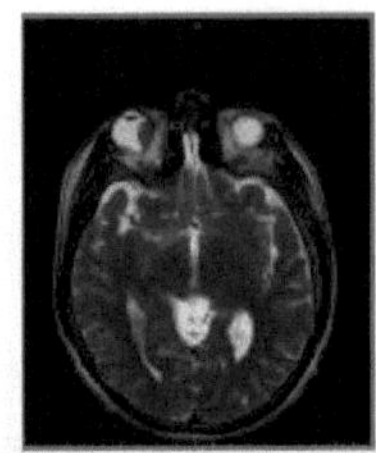

Fig. 19: Mélanome malin de la choroide de l'OD, a : signal hyper-intense en T1, b : signal hypo-intense en T2, A.Idder et al.

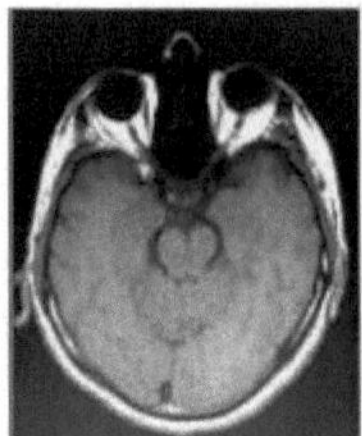 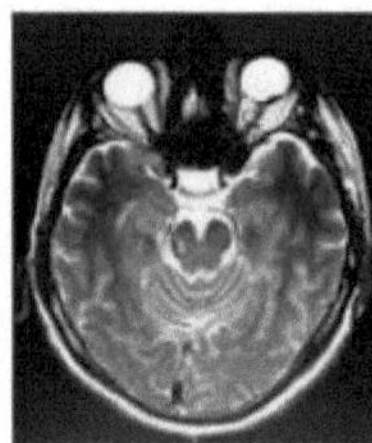 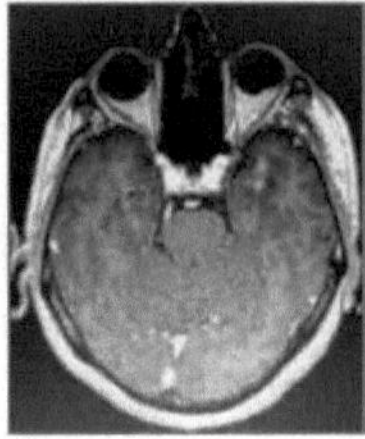

Fig. 20: Mélanome malin de la choroïde de l'OD, a : signal hyper-intense en T1, b : signal hypo-intense en T2, c rehaussement modéré après injection de gadolinium. Mesri. Kh

4.7. – Transillumination :

Transillumination can be used to detect or localize tumor margins. In general, pigmented tumors and intraocular hemorrhages block light transmission. Not all pigmented tumours are melanomas, and conversely, not all melanomas are pigmented (Fig. 21).

Various transillumination techniques :

—   Trans-pupillary, by placing the light source on the cornea. Care must be taken not to overestimate the posterior extension due to the shadow cast by an overly thick tumour.

—   Trans-ocular, with a transilluminator placed at right angles to the globe, diametrically opposite the tumor, less practical but more accurate than trans-pupillary.

—   Trans-scleral, with the light source on the sclera overhanging the tumor. This only determines whether the tumor transmits light or not.

Transillumination is also useful for identifying scleral necrosis and iris atrophy [44].

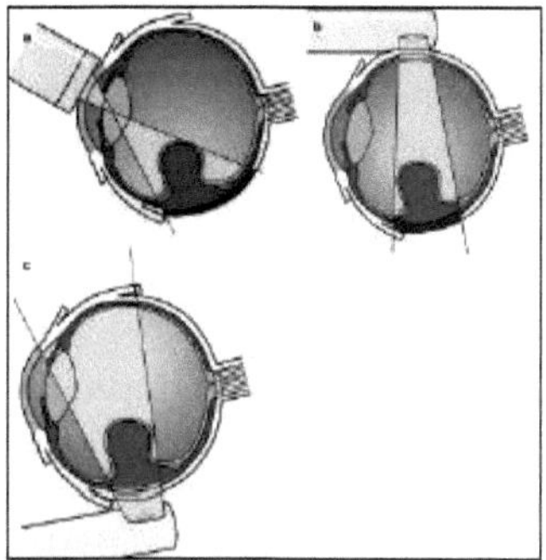

Fig. 21 : Techniques de transillumination. Extension tumorale évaluée par transillumination trans-pupillaire (a), transillumination trans-oculaire (b) et trans-sclérale (c). Notez l'exagération de l'extension postérieure de la tumeur avec transillumination transpupillaire [44]

Chapter V :
Results

We conducted a prospective descriptive study at the hospital specialized in ophthalmology (EHS) in Oran over a period of 18 years (2001- 2018).
The data collected concerned patients treated in the two ophthalmology departments A and B (Hammou Boutlélis clinic and Front de mer clinic).

1.   Caractéristiques Epidemiology of the study population:
1.1.   Répartition age by gender:

Patient age at diagnosis ranged from E=68 [17'85] years. The mean age was 53.7 ± 3.4 years, with a median of 54 years.
The modal age class is [50' 59] years, corresponding ta frequency of 30.2%.
The overall sex ratio was 0.9, showing a slight female predominance. In other words, for every 100 females, there were 90 males, except in the 30'39 and 40'49 age groups, where the ratio was 0.5 (Fig. 22).'

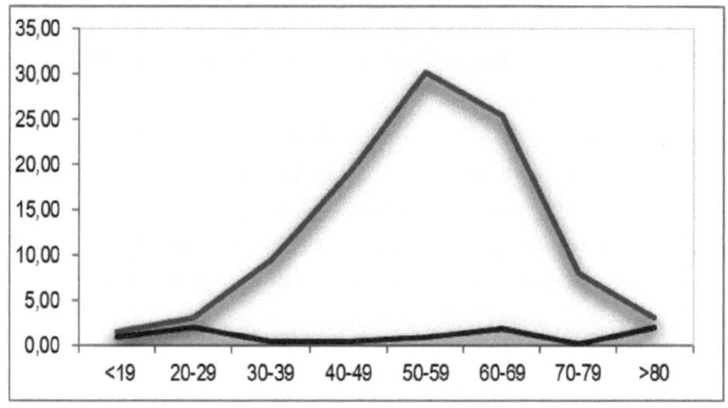

Fig. 22: Population distribution by age and sex ratio Oran ophthalmology hospital 2001 2018

1.2.   Etude phototype (skin color):

In our series, 50 patients (79.3%) were fair-skinned, 7 matt-skinned (11.1%), 4 very fair-skinned (6.3%), 1 dark-brown (1.6%), and only 1 melanoderm (1.6%)(Fig. 23).

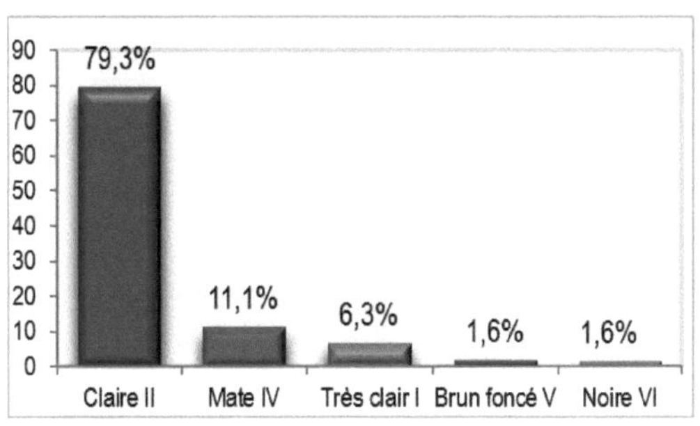

Patient phototype

Fig.23: Distribution of patients according to Fitzpatrick classification (by skin color) Oran ophthalmology hospital 2001 2018

1.3. Origine patient location:

Most patients were from western Algeria, with the wilaya of Oran origin first at 23.4%, followed by the wilaya of Tlemcen at 18.7% and the wilaya of Tiaret at 14% (Table II and Fig. 24).

Wilayas	Number of cases	%
Oran	15	23,8
Tlemcen	12	19,0
Tiaret	9	14,3
Relizane	7	11,1
Mascara	4	6,3
Sidi Bel Abbés	4	6,3
Mostaganem	2	3,2
Naama	2	3,2
Saïda	2	3,2
EChlef	1	1,6
Béchar	1	1,6
Sétif	1	1,6
Constantine	1	1,6
El Bayadh	1	1,6
Aïn Témouchent	1	1,6
Total	63	100

Table II: Geographical distribution of uveal melanoma cases in western Algeria Oran ophthalmology hospital 2001 2018

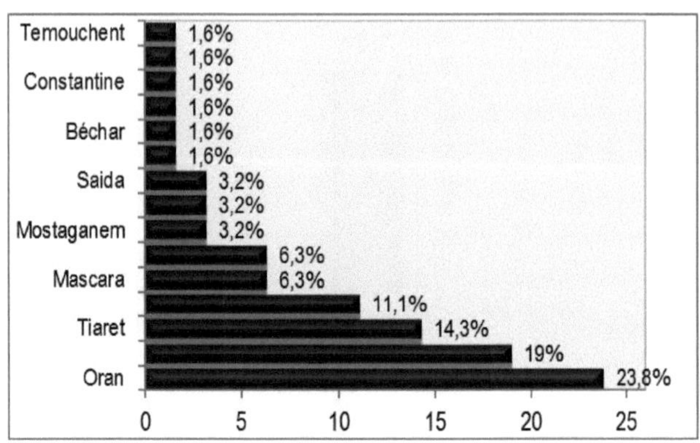

Number

Fig. 24: Geographical distribution of uveal melanomas
Oran ophthalmology hospital 2001‑2018

1.4. ꓸ Motif:

The main reason for consultation was reduced visual acuity in 34 patients (54%), followed by visual field amputation in 13 patients (20.6%). Uveal melanoma was discovered incidentally in 4 patients (6.3%), following ocular pain in 4 patients (6,3%), phosphenes in 3 patients (4.7%), myodesopsias in 2 patients (3.2%), paracentral scotoma in 1 patient (1.6%), and extra-scleral externalization in 1 patient (1.6%), and as part of the diagnosis of choroidal detachment after PKE in one patient (1.6% (Fig. 25).

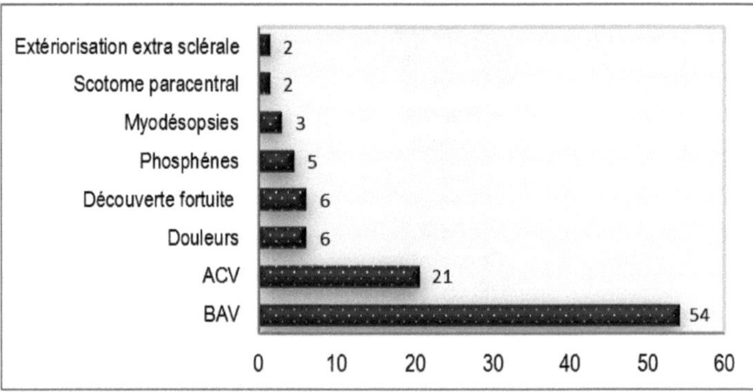

ACV: Amputation of the visual field BAV: Decrease in visual acuity

Fig.25: Main reasons for consultation Oran ophthalmology hospital 2001‑2018

2.   Caractéristiques clinical :
2.1.   Délais diagnostics:

Statistical characteristics of time to diagnosis	Statistical indicators
Range (in weeks) = $\varsigma\mu\alpha\xi$ – Vmin	96 0
Mean (in weeks) and 95% CI	12,3 [7,7 16,9]
Median (in weeks) and 95% CI	4,0 [4,0 – 8,0]
Standard deviation and Relative standard	18.0 and 146.2% for
Percentile P25 and IC95	3,0 [3,0 – 4,0]
Percentile P75 and IC95	12,0 [8,0 – 24,0]
Agost test ino-Pearson for ıtion normal	(P 0,0001) Rejection of normality test
(efficient d'asyn ét e or skewne ss	2,8 (P 0,0001)
(efficient de kur ose or kurtosis or solidissement	8,7 (P 0,0001)

Table III: Principal summary statistical characteristics of time to diagnosis of uveal melanoma - EHS ophthalmology Oran 2001 2018

00

Diagnosis time (in weeks)

In 48.4% of our population, it is ≤ 4 weeks after the onset of the first symptoms (N=30), with an average duration of 3.4 weeks.
ı In 33.8% of cases, it varies from 5 24 weeks
ı In 8% of cases, it ranged from 25 weeks to 1 year, and more than 1 year in 3.2%. In 4 of our patients, the diagnosis was made during a routine examination (6.3%) (Table IV); the mean time to diagnosis was 12.3 weeks or 3 months, with a median of 4 weeks.
It should be noted that one patient with a diagnostic delay of over 10 years could not be included in the data analysis.

Deadlines (weeks)	Number	%
0 4	34	54,8
5 7	0	0
8 24	21	33,8
25 48	5	8
≥ 72	2	3,2
Total	62	100

Table IV: Diagnostic time in weeks Oran ophthalmology hospital 2001 2018

2.2. Latéralité of the tumor:

The uveal melanoma was located on the OD in 32 patients (50.8%), and on the left side in 31 patients (49.2%) OD/OG laterality ratio 1.03.

2. 3. Acuité visual at the time of diagnosis :

Visual acuity at the time of diagnosis of uveal melanoma averaged 1.1 Log MAR, or around 9/100 in decimal values, ranging from negative light perception (PL·) to 10/10.

2.4. Vascularisation sentinel:

Episcleral sentinel vascularization was present in 42 patients (66.6%), absent in 13 patients (20.6%), unspecified in 7 patients (11.1%), and not visible in one patient (1.6%), for its location (Fig. 26). In terms of location, it was nasal in 11 patients (26.2%), temporal in 6 patients (14.3%), inferior temporal in 6 patients (14.3%), inferior in 5 patients (12.0%), temporal in 4 patients (9.5%), superior nasal in 4 patients (9.5%), inferior nasal in 3 patients (7.1%), sentinel vascularization superior in one patient (1.6%), nasal with externalization in one patient (1.6%), superior temporal in one patient (1.6%) and inferior in one patient (1.6%)(N=42)(Fig. 27).

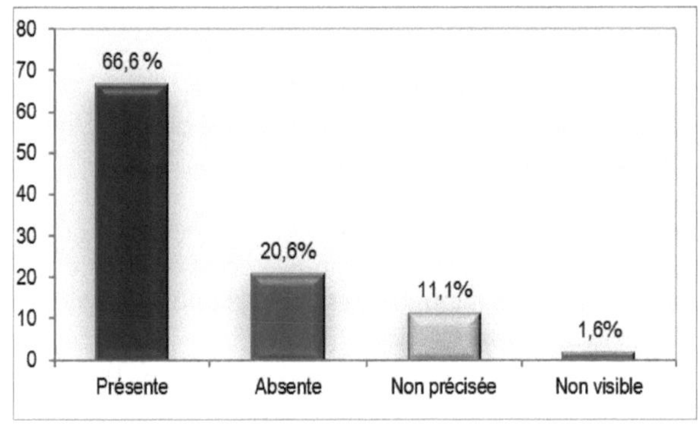

Fig. 26: Sentinel vasculature EHS ophthalmologie d'Oran 2001 2018

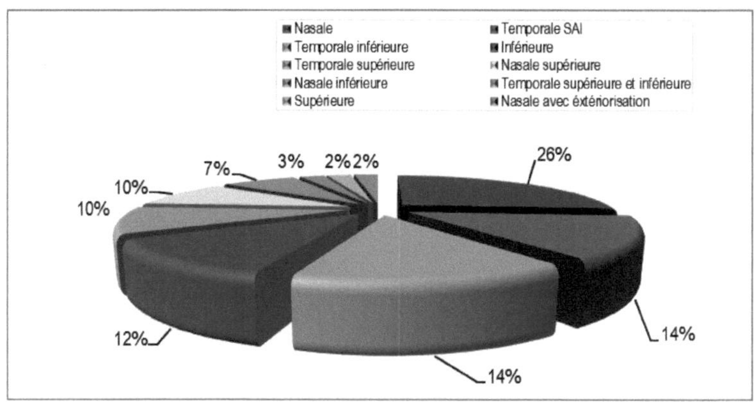

Fig. 27: Site of sentinel vascularization EHS ophthalmologie d'Oran 2001 2018

2.5. Couleur of the iris:

We note that 44 patients had brown irises (70%), 9 green irises (14.3%), 8 light brown (12.7%), 2 blue (3.2%) (Fig. 28).

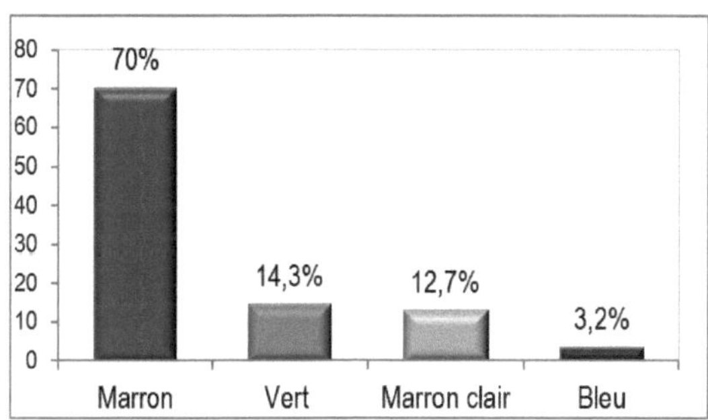

Iris color

Fig. 28: Iris color of patients with uveal melanoma EHS ophthalmology
Oran 2001 2018

2.6. Lésions melanin :

The absence of melanic lesions in 44 patients (70%), iridial nevi were present on ODG in 12 patients (19%), pigmented lesions of the FO in 4 patients (6.3%), choroidal nevus in one patient, pigment dispersion on the iris in one patient, and a combination of iridial and cutaneous nevi in one patient, i.e. 1.6% (Fig. 29).

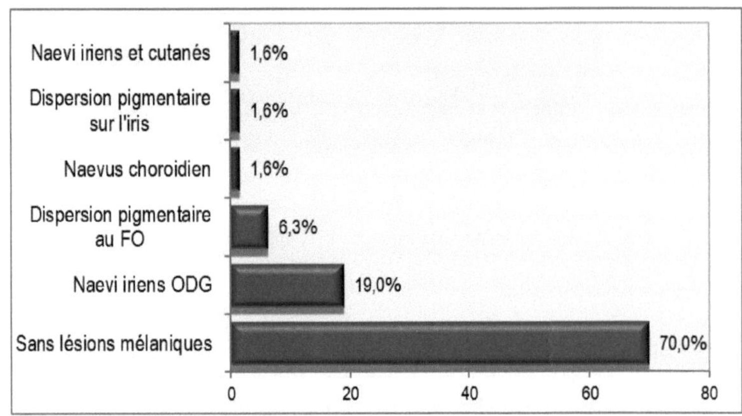

Fig. 29: Melanoma lesions in patients with uveal melanoma EHS ophthalmologie d'Oran 2001 2018

2.7. Siège:

In our series 62 patients had choroidal melanoma (98.4%), one patient had melanoma of the ciliary body (1.6%).35 patients (55.5%) hadchoroidal melanoma in the equatorial region, 9 patients (14.3%) in the posterior pole, 6 patients (9.5%) in the parapapapillary region, 6 patients (9.5%) in the preequatorial region.

in 6 patients (9.5%) occupying the entire cavity in 4 patients (6.3%), annular in 2 patients (3.2%) (Fig. 30).

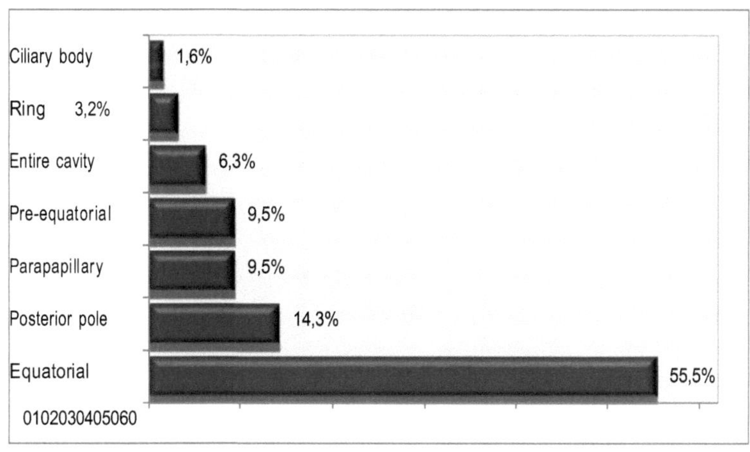

Frequency

Fig. 30: Site of uveal melanoma EHS ophthalmology Oran 2001 2018

Pigmentation melanoma: pigmented neoformation in 55 patients (87.3%), achrome in 6 patients (9.5%), and heterogeneous in 2 patients (3.2%) (Fig. 31)

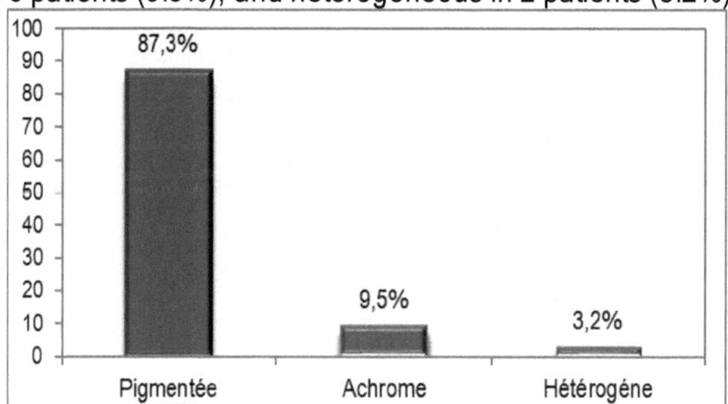

Neoformation pigmentation

Fig. 31: Pigmentation of the EHS ophthalmology neoformation in Oran 2001 2018

2.8. Décollement of secondary retina and serous retinal detachment:

Secondary retinal detachment (DR II) was present in 22 patients or 35%, while serous retinal detachment (SRD) was present in 21 patients or 33.3%(Fig. 32).

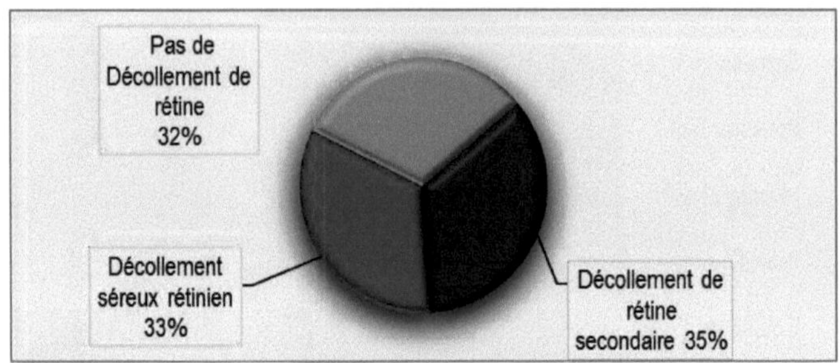

Fig. 32: Secondary retinal detachment and serous retinal detachment associated with uveal melanoma EHS ophthalmologie d'Oran 2001 2018

3. Caractéristiques ultrasonography :

3.1. Excavation and ultrasound attenuation: Choroidal excavation was present in 57 patients or 90.5%, ultrasound attenuation was high in 57 patients (90.5%), low in 5 patients (8%), and average in one patient (1.6%) (Fig. 33).

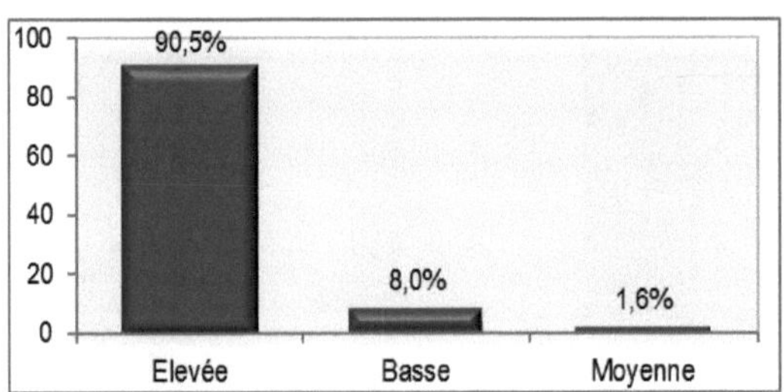

Ultrasound attenuation

Fig. 33: Ultrasound attenuation by uveal melanoma EHS ophthalmology Oran 2001 2018

3.2. Forme of neoformation :

The neoformation was dome-shaped in 29 patients (46%), rounded in 25 patients (39.7%), mushroom-shaped in 7 patients (11.1%), shirt button-shaped in one patient (1.6%), ring-shaped in only one case (1.6%) (Fig. 34).

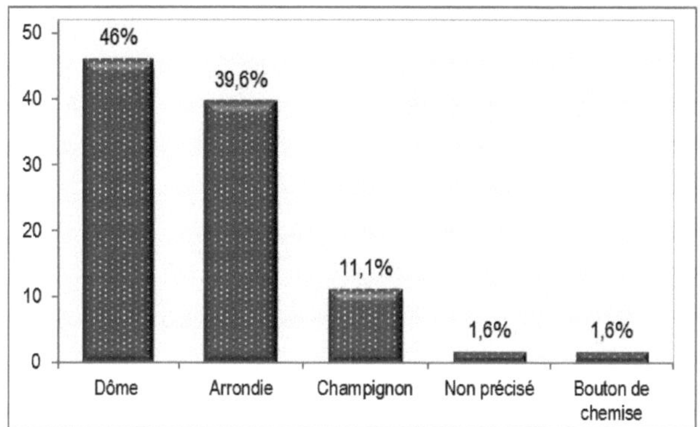

Form of neoformation

Fig. 34: Shape of the EHS ophthalmology neoformation in Oran 2001 2018

3.3. Taille and tumor thickness:

Tumor measurements taken by B-mode ultrasound, and Echodoppler, with 10 and 15Mhz probes. The largest basal diameter (LDB) was ≤ 10mm in 23 patients (36.5%), this diameter was >10mm in 39 patients (62%). Tumor PGD ranged from [4.0·18.3] mm, with a mean of 11.2 mm. Tumor thickness was≤5 mm in 10 patients (15.8%), >5 mm in 51 patients (81%), but remained unspecified in 3.2%. Tumor thickness ranged from [1.61·16.8] mm. The mean thickness was 8 mm (Fig. 35 ,36).

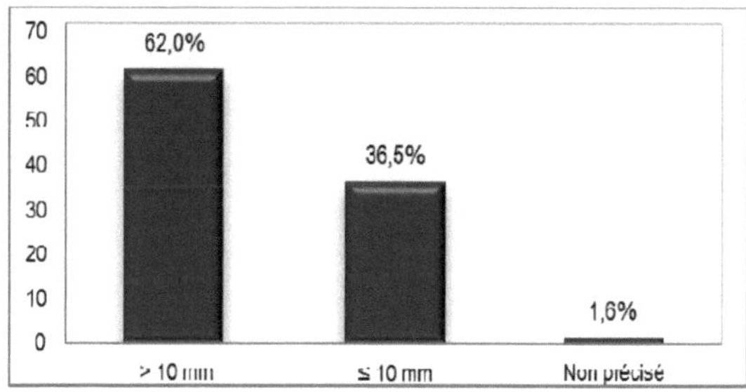

PGD

Fig. 35 : Diamètre du mélanome uvéal
EHS ophtalmologie d'Oran 2001–2018

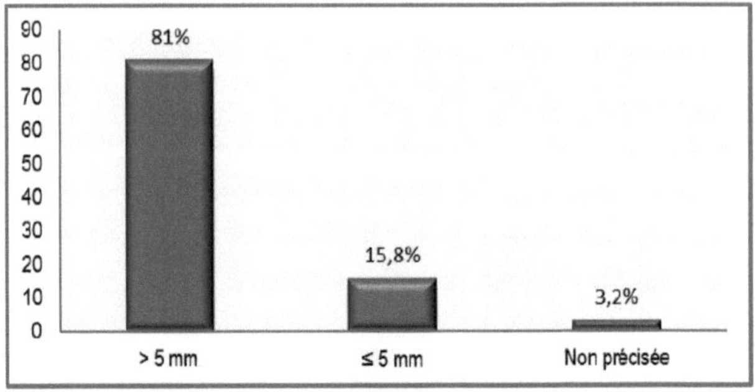

Epaisseur tumorale

Fig. 36: Epaisseur du mélanome uvéal
EHS ophtalmologie d'Oran 2001–2018

4.   Ⅰ Classification TNM :

Depending on the size, tumor extension and location of the mass. In our series, 49 tumors were classified T_3 (77.7%), 8 T_2 (12.7%), 2 T_4 (3.2%), T_{1a} (1.6%) and T_{1b} one case (1.6%), unspecified for one tumor (1.6%), and finally one ciliary body tumor classified T_3 (1.6%).

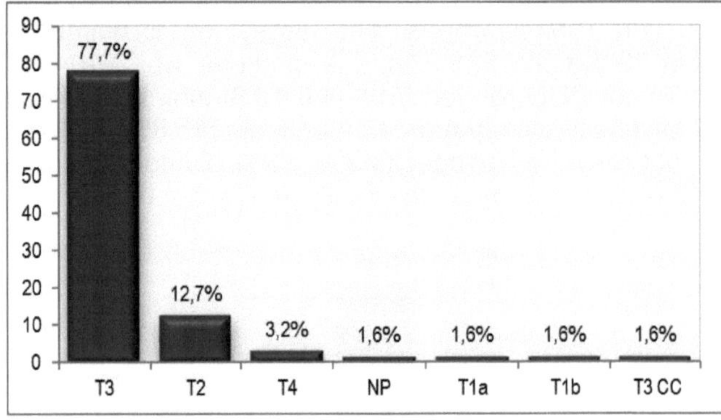

TNM classification
Fig. 37: TNM classification of uveal melanomas
Oran ophthalmology hospital 2001Ⅰ 2018

5. | **OCT (optical coherence tomography) macular:**Macular OCT revealed DSR in 2 patients (15.4%), DSR+ deposits on the outer surface of the raised retina in 5 patients (38.4%), MEM in 2 patients (15.4%), OMC in 2 patients (15.4%), intravitreal hemorrhage interfering with the examination in one patient, normal macular profile in 2 patients(15.4%), the examination was not performed in 49 patients (N=13) (Fig. 38)

6. | **Echodoppler ocular:** using a 15 Mhz probe, the examination was performed in 11 patients (17.4%), including 1 patient with a richly vascularized mass (9%), 6 with moderate vascularization (54.5%), 3 with poor vascularization (27.2%), and one mass that was avascular (9%) (Fig. 39).

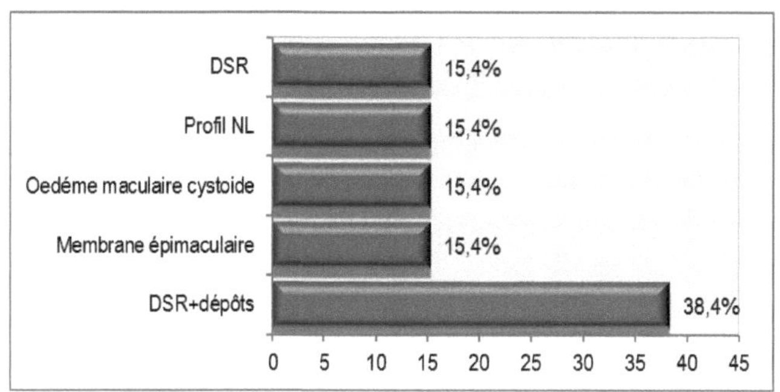

Fig.38: Macular OCT of uveal melanomas
Oran ophthalmology hospital 2001| 2018

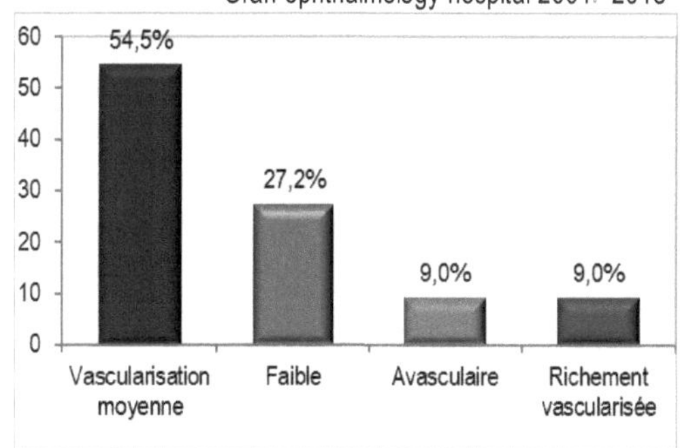

Vascularization of the neoformation

Fig. 39: Tumor vascularization using color Doppler Bounoua.C
vascular surgeon
Oran ophthalmology hospital 2001| 2018

1. Aspects epidemiological :

1.1. Fréquence :

The incidence of uveal melanoma depends on the race and demographic profile of the population [3,68].

Our study, which covered a period of 18 years, collected 63 cases of uveal melanoma, an average of 3 cases per year, very few figures exist on anational scale, we only found a study carried out by a team from the BLIDA Faculty of Sciences at CHU Mustapha which reported, 40 cases of uveal melanoma over a period of 11 years [2005-2015], with an average of 3.6 cases per year [Si mahdi.H, Tabbouche.N 2015].

Our figures are similar to those of our Tunisian neighbors, who over a 23-year period diagnosed 80 cases of uveal melanoma, or 3.5 cases per year [1990-2013] [69].

Very few figures are available in Algeria, on the incidence of uveal melanoma. During 2014, 5 MU were diagnosed out of 19,000 (0.026%) consultations in the emergency department of Oran's specialized ophthalmology hospital, in China at the ophthalmology clinic of Shanghai's First Medical College, the rate was 4.5 MU per 10,000 (0.045%) hospitalized patients [23].

Authors and references	Period	Period	Country
Ischovich et al. 1995	1961-1989	0,57	Israel
Vidal et al. 1995 [155]	1992	0,73	France
Virgili et al. 2007 [156]	1983-1994	<0.2 Spain and Italy >0.8 Norway and Denmark	Europe
Singh	1973-2008	0.58 male, 0.44 woman	United States
Kricker	1996-1998	0.11 male, 0.78 woman	Australia
Bergman	1960-1998	0, 4 men, 0.88 woman	Sweden

Table V: Incidence of uveal melanoma in the world population, number of cases per 100,000 inhabitants. Adapted from [3,44] EHS ophtalmologie d'Oran 2001 2018

1.2. Age and gender:

In our study, the average age of patients with uveal melanoma was 53.7±3.4 years, a figure corresponding to the average age in the 1950s [3], with an increase in the number of cases from the age of 40 onwards. According to Zografos et al. 2002 [3], the average age was estimated at 62 years, with incidence increasing from the fourth decade and peaking in the 6th and 7th, with a fall in incidence in the over-80 age groups. Damato.B [44] from 1973 and 1997, speaks of an incidence rate that peaked in the 7th decade.

The average age of patients who develop uveal melanoma has progressively increased over the last 50 years, with the median age at diagnosis of uveal melanoma being 59 to 62 years [11,12,13].

In a study of epidemiological trends in uveal melanoma among 7043 patients in the SEER (The Surveillance, Epidemiology, and End Results in the USA) database from 1973 to 2009, the mean age at diagnosis increased between 1973 (59 years) and 2009 (62 years) [13]. In our series, over an 18-year period, the most affected age bracket was [18,28], i.e. the fifth decade, with a total of 19 patients (30%), and 2 patients over 80 years of age (3.1%), the COMS study (Collaborative OcularMelanomaStudy), which lasted 11.5 years from 1986 to 1998 and involved 43 centers across the USA and Canada, with 1317 patients, found 268 cases in the [50-59] bracket, and 408 cases in the [29,39] bracket, i.e. the 6th decade (31%), and 4.2% of patients were over 80 years of age; our patients are around 10 years younger at the time of diagnosis, as are Asians and Saudis [70,71], compared with the white North American population [3, 13, 72] (Fig. 40).

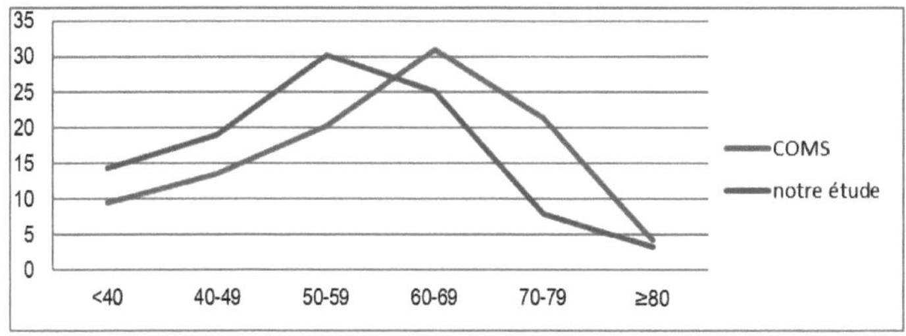

Fig. 40: Comparison of age groups affected by MU between the COMS study and our own.

Uveal melanoma is exceptional before puberty. Singh et al [7] found 63 cases of uveal melanoma in adolescents under 20 years of age out of 8,000 diagnosed cases (0.8%); in our study, this rate was 1.6%. Zografos et al [3], Windsor.S et al [18] report a slight male predominance of around 5%, while this predominance remains debatable for other authors Singh et al [12] and the COMS 2001 study [72]. In our case series, there were 33 women and 30 men, with a sex ratio of 0.9.

1.3. Race :

Data in the literature on the incidence of uveal melanoma in different ethnic groups and races show that incidence is inversely proportional to the degree of skin pigmentation. They also suggest that melanoma develops at a younger age in melanodermal people than in the Caucasian population, according to Zografos et al. [3] Uveal melanomas mainly affect the Caucasian race; in highly pigmented individuals, the incidence is low. A review of the literature shows that only 10 patients of African race were among the 3586 cases treated for melanoma

(0.3%) at the Wills EyeHospital in Philadelphia between 1974 and 1989, and only 8 of the 1527 patients enucleated for melanoma in the COMS study between 1996 and 1998 (0.5%) were African-Americans [3]. On the African continent, 1 case of melanoma among 164 ocular and orbital tumors treated between 1962 and 1992 (0.6%) at the Congo-Kinshasa ophthalmology clinic [20], in South Africa, Miller et al, found 1 case of melanoma in a native patient compared with 153 cases in the Caucasian population during the same observation period (1954-1978), with an estimated ratio of 1:80 [21],Malik and Sheikh in Sudan found 6 cases of uveal melanoma among 854 tumours of the eye and adnexa (0.7%), in the Arab part of the population [22], [3].

The incidence of uveal melanoma is low in patients with intermediate pigmentation: Asians, North Africans, Latin Americans, and Indo-Americans, in China at the ophthalmology clinic of the first medical college in Shanghai, 65 cases of melanoma were treated between 1956-1975, melanoma appeared to develop at a younger age than in the Caucasian race Cunningham, Mann.Kuo et al., [23] Incidence is also low in the Middle East, such as Iran, Afghanistan and India [3]. In Israel, the incidence of uveal melanoma is higher in Jews of European or American origin, compared with Jews of African or Asian origin, underlining the relationship between uveal melanoma incidence and degrees of skin pigmentation [3].

No statistical difference in metastasis or death by MU according to ethnic origin has been reported [73].

The Algerian population is of intermediate pigmentation, according to Fitzpatrick's classification for the different phototypes, most of our patients were fair-skinned, 50 patients or 79.3%, 7 matt (11.1%), 4 very dark-skinned (11.1%), and 1 very dark-skinned (11.1%).

light (6.3%), 1 dark brown (1.6%), and 1 melanoderm (1.6%)

Interestingly, with regard to age and race, our population seems to be affected at a younger age than the Caucasian race, in line with the results found in different ethnic groups, with intermediate pigmentation, in Africa and Asia.

In 2007, the EUROCARE (European Cancer Registry) working group studied the distribution of 6673 MU between 1983 and 1994 in 16 European countries at different latitudes [154].In Spain and southern Italy, the incidence rate of MU was less than two cases per million, while in Norway and Denmark, the incidence rate was more than eight cases per million [164]. A 10° latitude difference was marked by an increase in MU incidence, The decreasing north-south gradient supports the protective role ocular pigmentation; there is a 4° latitude difference between Algeria (36°) and Spain (40°), which could explain the differences in incidence between the North African and European populations. A 4° latitude difference between northern and southern Algeria, Oran 35°, Bechar 31°, Tiaret 35°, Tlemcen 34°.

1.4.   Origine patient location:

Most patients were from the wilaya of Oran (23.8%), Tlemcen (19%) and Tiaret (14.3%), Relizane (11.1%), Mechria (3.2%), El-Bayadh (1.6%), Bechar (1.6%),

Wilayas	Latitudes	of patients affected
Oran	35°41'	23,8
Tlemcen	34°52'	19,0
Tiaret	34°52'	14,3
Relizane	35°44'	11,1
Mechria	33°16'	3,2
El bayadh	33°41'	1,6
Bechar	31°37'	1,6

Table VI: Distribution of patients by latitude of wilayas οριγινε– EHS ophthalmologie d'Oran 2001 2018

Indeed, we found a statistically significant correlation between light phototype and geographical origin (p=0.001), with 75% of light phototype patients living in northern cities, with high latitude, the decreasing north-south gradient would support the protective role of skin pigmentation.

2. Facteurs risk :

2.1. Couleur of the iris:

Multiple studies in Canada, the USA, Germany, France and Australia have shown that MU has a higher incidence in people with light irises [74,75]. Other studies argue more for an association with skin type [74], but it is difficult to separate the two. In addition, an association between the risk of metastatic death from MU and blue or grey iris has been found [76].

Some researchers suggest that the reason why a dark iris color leads to a lower risk of developing MU than a light iris color, is due to the protective role of the higher percentage of melanin in dark eyes [77].

Houtzagers, L et al at Leiden University Medical Center in the Netherlands, of 412 eyes enucleated for MU, 65% had blue/grey eyes, 16% brown iris, intermediate color (green or hazel) in 19%, Leiden cohort [78].

In our series, 44 patients had brown irises (70%), 17 irises of intermediate color (green and or hazel) or 27%, 2 blue (3.2%).

Our figures are the reverse of Leiden University's figures for browns and greys/blues.

2.2. Facteurs exogenous risk :

Exposure to the sun and to artificial UV rays, professions at risk are mainly represented by arc welders, and professional cooks [41,42], these risk factors have not been studied in our case series.

Harbour.JW et al, [78], hypothesized that darker choroidal pigmentation could represent a response to higher levels of chronic UV irradiation. In support of this, Li.W et al established a correlation between light iris and posterior location of uveal melanoma. They demonstrated that tumor distribution correlated with the distribution of light rays on the posterior segment, and that the macular and perimacular region was more exposed to UV radiation, in light irises, in our study, 2 patients presented very light-colored irises, and melanomas of the posterior pole (photo 12).

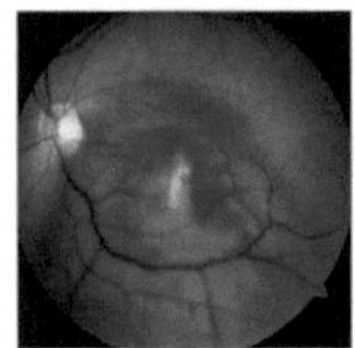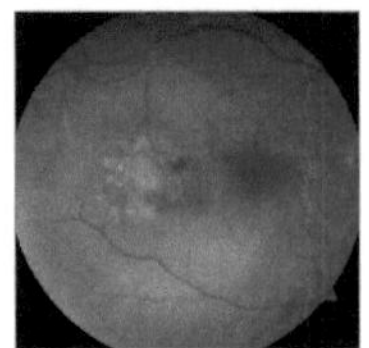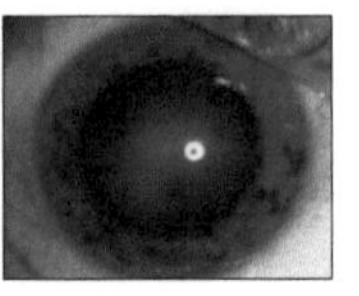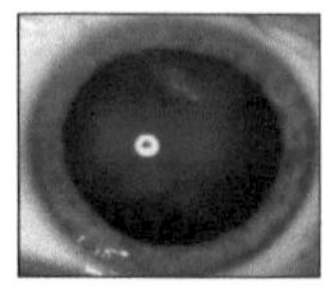

Photo 12: Melanomas of the posterior pole in patients with clear irises, EHS Ophtalmologie d'Oran

3. Aspects clinical :

3.1. Motif:

The main reason for consultation was decreased visual acuity, reported by most authors, Zografos et al [3] 48.8%, 42% for Chebbi et al [38], and 54% for our series, visual field amputation represented 20.6%, in our series, and 16% for Ah-fat.FG, Damato et al. myodesopsias represented 3.2% in our study and 4% for Ah-fat.FG, Damato et al. [79], our figures are close to those in the literature.

Asymptomatic MU accounted for 28% in Damato et al. and 10% in Zografos et al. and 6.3% in our series. These variations may be due to differences in diagnostic modalities between departments.

3.2. Délai diagnostic :

Chebbi et al [6], in a series of 80 cases, found an average delay in diagnosis of 6.8 months, with extremes of 1-36 months; in our study, the average delay was 3 months, with extremes of 1-24 months.G and Damato.B [79], in a series of 50 patients, observed over a 4-month period, at the Liverpool Ocularoncology service during 1996, 58% of patients were diagnosed after an average of 4.2 weeks, and 42% were diagnosed after an average of 6.6 months, 6 of whom were seen by an optometrist, 3 by a general practitioner, 4 were misdiagnosed as benign nevi or AMD, 3 had been mistaken for suspicious nevi, 1 patient misplaced his referral letter, 1 patient was followed up for MEM, and 3 others were diagnosed with MMC, but only followed up, in our study 47.6% of patients were diagnosed before 01 months, and 8% after 6 months, a lower percentage than that of Damato et al. This epidemiological characteristic (delay in diagnosis) appears very rarely in studies of uveal melanoma, which could mean that in other oculo-oncology centers, diagnosis is made earlier than in our study (access to care).

3.3 Latéralité :

Choroidal melanoma has been diagnosed with similar frequency in both eyes, right and left in most authors [72], in our study, DO involvement accounted for 50.8%, against 48.2% for the OG.

3.4 Acuité visual at time of diagnosis:

If we compare our VAs with those of Diener.W et al in the COMS study(Fig. 41), our visual acuities are lower at the time of diagnosis: 65% of patients had a VA ≤ 2/10, compared with 16.9% of patients in the COMS study, and only 9.5% of patients had a VA ≥ 10/10, compared with 31.3% (the highest percentage) in the COMS study, In the COMS study, more than 2/3 of patients were treated less than a month after diagnosis.

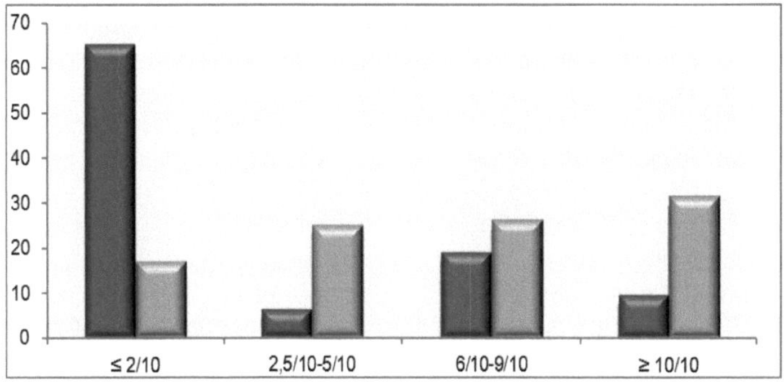

Fig. 41: Comparison of VAs between our patient series and the COMS study.

3.5. Vascularisation sentinel:

Sentinel vascularization was present in 66.6% of patients in our series, compared with 3.5% of patients in the COMS 2001 study [72], and absent in 20.6% of patients in our series, compared with 96.5% in the COMS study.4% of tumors had a thickness ≤ 5 mm for the COMS, and 81% of our tumors had a thickness > 5mm, episcleral vascularization was not mentioned in 7 patients (11.1%), and not visible in one patient (1.6%), since he presented an extra scleral externalization of his choroidal melanoma in our series of patients.

In our study, we found a statistically significant correlation between sentinel vascularization and tumor PGD (p=0.005), with 42% of patients with sentinel vascularization having a PGD>10mm.

3.6. Lésions melanin :

Concerning pigment dispersions in the FO, Lahav.M et al. [80], examining 54 eyeballs with MMC, 28 tumors were of the spindle-shaped type, 24 of the mixed type, and two of the epithelioid type, found that in 80% of the tumors studied, pigment-laden cells had accumulated far from the tumor region and at the periphery of the sub-retinal space, the dispersion of tumour cells is mainly observed in melanomas of the epithelioid type[3], in our study, for enucleated patients, one patient presented a pigment dispersion on the iris (photo 13), this was an epithelioid melanoma, and two others with pigment dispersions on the FO (photo 14), one was of mixed type, and the other of undetermined histological type.

Melanoma lesions were absent in 44 patients (70%), with fusiform melanoma accounting for 64.5% in our series, which could explain the relatively low rate of pigment dispersion, which is more frequent in the epithelioid type.

Irial nevi are recognized as a risk factor for uveal melanoma in general, and iris melanoma in particular [77], in our series,

12 patients had iris nevi (19%), patients with cutaneous nevi have a 4.36 to 10.4 times greater risk of developing uveal melanoma than the general population [77], in our study 2 patients had cutaneous nevi, including one who had both (cutaneous and iris nevi), and who died of liver metastases.

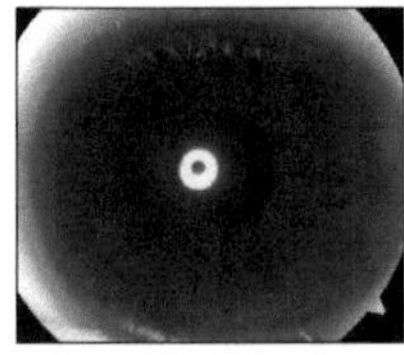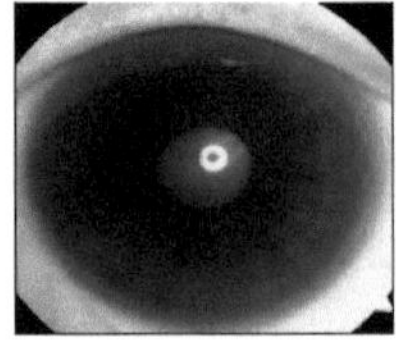

Photo 13: 2 eyes of the same patient, a) OD pigment dispersion on the iris surface, b) OG, note the difference in iris surface in ODG EHS Ophthalmology of Oran

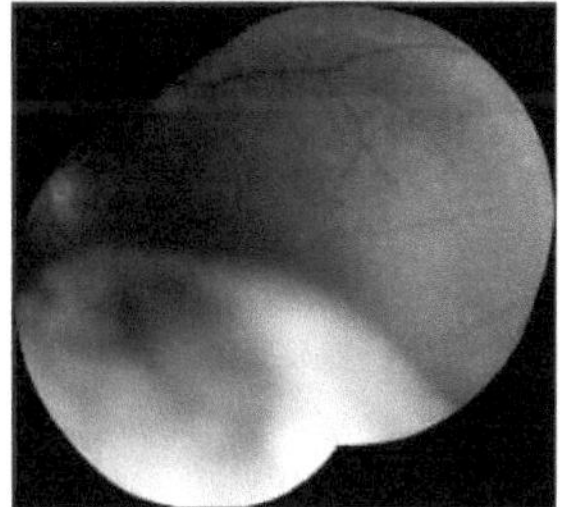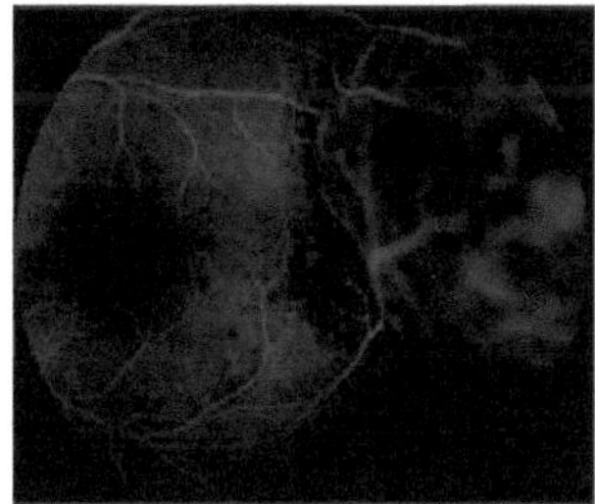

Photo 14 : Dispersion pigmentaire au FO, à distance et à proximité de la tumeur. EHS Ophtalmologie d'Oran

Photo 14: Pigment dispersion in the FO, at a distance and close to the tumor. EHS Ophthalmology of Oran

3.7. Siège of the mass :

The starting point of 80-90% of intraocular melanomas is the choroid [3,44], Chebbi et al [6] had 90% MMC and 3.7% ciliary body melanomas, in our case series, choroidal melanoma accounted for 98.4%, and the ciliary body 1.6%, our results are similar to those reported in the literature. Regarding tumor location (Fig. 42), in our series, the equatorial location was the most frequent, unlike Chebbi. A et al, for whom the pre-equatorial location was the most frequent, as well as involvement of the posterior pole, which was more important than in our study, 4 of our patients presented with melanomas occupying the entire cavity, for Chebbi. A et al had 5 patients.

In the COMS study by Diener.W et al, more than half the patients had posterior pole melanomas, probably related to the light iris color of most patients.

In our case series, melanomas of the posterior pole accounted for 14.3%, which could be linked to the protective role of iris pigmentation, since more than 2/3 of patients have brown irises and are of intermediate pigmentation [69].

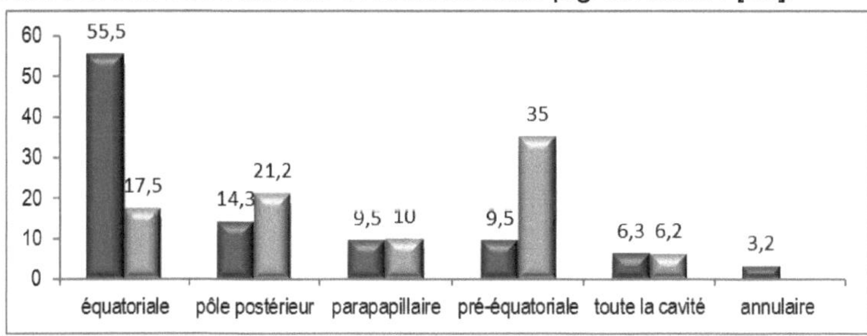

Fig. 42: Location of choroideal melanomas, our series and Chebbi's. A et al.

3.8. Pigmentation of neoformation: according to Kalili.S and Shields.CL [77], 55% of melanomas are pigmented, 15% are achromic, and 30% heterogeneous, in our study, pigmented melanomas represented 87.3%,

achromic 9.5%, and heterogeneous 3.2%, one might think that this high rate of pigmented melanomas could be related to the study population, which in our case, is of intermediate pigmentation, but interestingly, 67.2% of pigmented melanomas are associated with light phototype, so there is no correlation between tumor pigmentation and patient phototype. Harbour et al [69] had found that dark choroidal pigmentation was a risk factor for the development of uveal melanoma in the Caucasian population, in relation to chronic UV exposure, which could explain our results.

The degree of iris pigmentation is a consequence of both the total melanin content of the epithelial cells and stromal melanocytes, and the proportion of two different types of melanin: Eumelanin, found in dark-skinned individuals, is more photo-protective, This pigmentation is essential for controlling pupil aperture and, perhaps, for UV filtration, as in the case of the skin. On the other hand, this pigmentation could be a risk factor in the development of choroidal melanoma in white patients. This finding may have implications for understanding the pathogenesis of uveal melanoma [69,32].

Dark choroidal pigmentation may present a higher risk of oxidative DNA damage in choroidal melanocytes, compared to lighter choroidal pigmentation [69], as melanin is a photoactive element and can paradoxically act as a photo-sensitizer or photo-protector.

Our study population is characterized by dark iris and choroidal pigmentation, in a country where solar radiation is high, which would support the idea of the protective role of iris pigmentation, loaded with Eumelanin absorbing a large amount of UV, thus reducing DNA damage to choroidal melanocytes and consequently the total number duveal melanomas in our population compared to light pigmented populations.

3.9. Forme of neoformation :

Half of our melanomas were dome-shaped (Fig. 43), and 12.6% shirt-button-shaped. In the COMS study [72], dome-shaped melanomas accounted for 77%, and shirt-button-shaped melanomas for 16%; in Chebbi. A et al [6], dome-shaped melanomas represented 54%, and shirt-button 24%, our figures agree with the COMS for the shirt-button shape, and the Tunisian study for the dome shape, thus confirming the data in the literature.

39.7% of our patients have a rounded tumor shape. According to Zografos et al, the rounded shape is linked to a homogeneous distribution of mitoses [3].

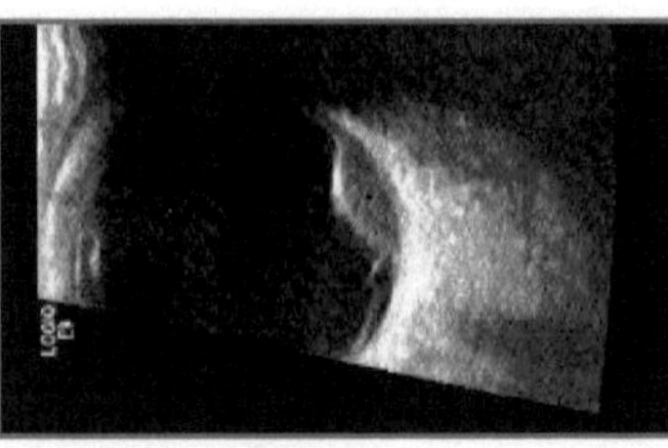
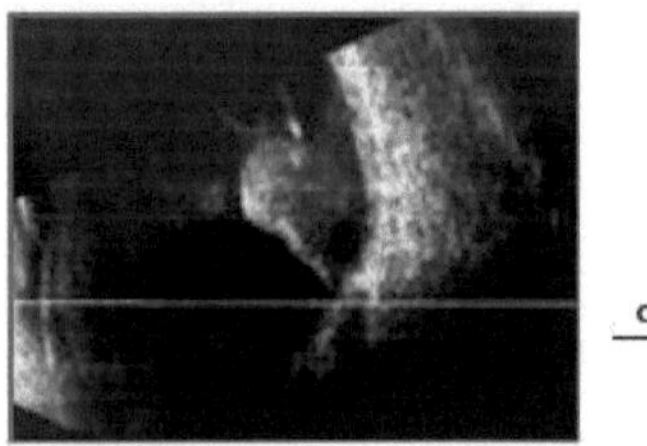

Fig. 43 : Néoformations avec DR secondaire a) en dôme, b) en champignon EHS ophtalmologie d'Oran, et Bounoua.C

3.10. Décollement retinal detachment II area: choroidal melanoma is almost always accompanied by secondary retinal detachment [44]; in our study, DR was associated with neoformation in 68% of cases, for COMS
[72] Secondary DR was present in 55% of patients (photo 15).

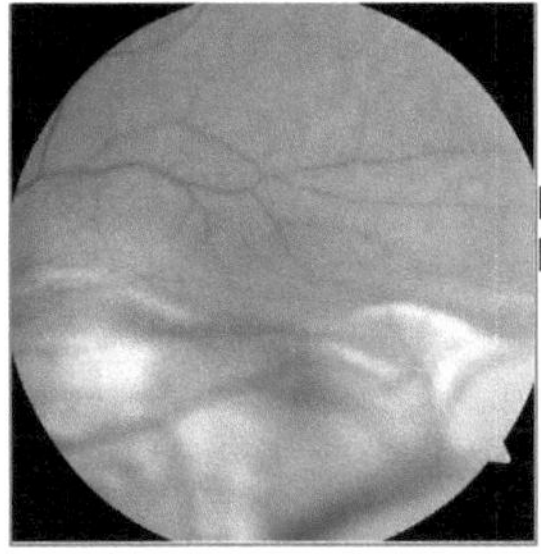

Photo 15: Neoformation associated with secondary DR, EHS ophthalmology Oran

3.11. Excavation choroidal: present in 90.5%, for COMS 84%, in line with literature data.

3.12. Taille and tumor thickness: 15.8% of our patients had a tumor thickness ≤ 5mm, versus 30% for Chebbi et al. 45% of patients had a thickness ≤4mm for COMS, with an average of 4.8mm, 81% of our tumors had a thickness >5mm, versus 69% for Chebbi et al., this would mean that our tumors are thicker, with an average of 8mm. The tumoral PGD (largest diameter) was >10mm in 62%, versus 80% for Chebbi et al [6], it was ≤10mm in 36.5% of our patients, versus 20% for Chebbi et al, the mean tumoral PGD was 11.2mm in our study, that of COMS [72] was 11.4mm, our tumors had a tumor PGD, on average, lower than that of Tunisians and about the same as that of Americans, in other words, our tumors are thicker but less wide. The thickness of dome-shaped melanomas is equal to half the tumor diameter. If Bruch's lamina ruptures, this sub-retinal part escapes the mechanical constraints of this lamina, and will have a spherical shape.

[3] (photo 16), which is the case for 39.7% of our patients, we would have more cases of Bruch's blade rupture if compared with other studies.

27% of our patients developed liver metastases, 59% of them with rounded melanomas, 11.7% with mushroom-shaped melanomas and 29% with domed melanomas, confirming that rupture of Bruch's membrane is a poor prognostic factor.

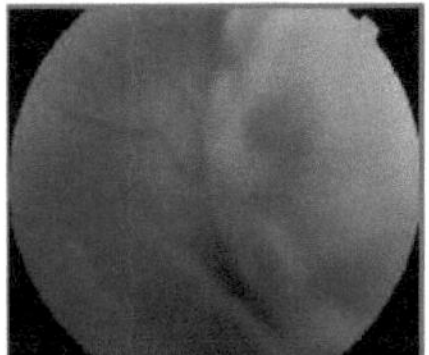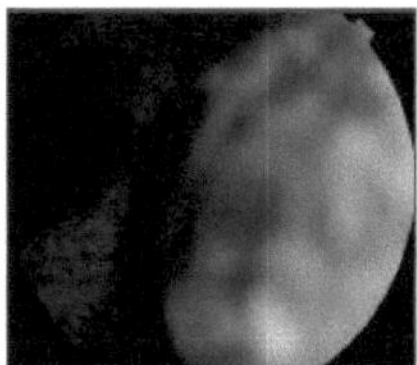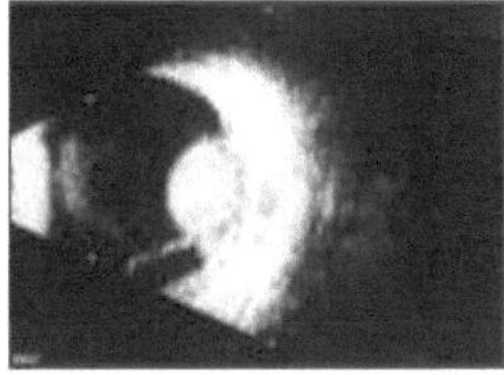

Photo 16 : Mélanome malin de la choroide, arrondie avec DR secondaire, a : photo du FO couleur, b ; séquence angiographique, c : échographie en mode B.
EHS ophtalmologie d'Oran

3.13. Classification TNM :

Shields CL et al [81], based on the American Joint Committee on Cancer (AJCC) 7th edition tumor classification, on 7731 patients, found, stage I 36%, stage II 48%, stage III 16%, stage IV < 1%, in our case series, based on clinical and ultrasound data, the highest percentage was stage III 77.7%, stage II 12.7%, stage IV 3.2%, stage I 3.2%, for Chebbi et al [6], the highest percentage was stage IV, 32.5%, and a more or less even distribution for the other stages, with stage I at 21.3%. What we can conclude, and what has been said above, is that our tumors are larger at the time of diagnosis, compared with the American study, probably due to a delay in diagnosis, but much smaller than the Tunisian study (Fig. 44).

> UICC (International Union Against Cancer) TNM classification of choroid and ciliary body melanomas, adapted from [3].
> For melanoma of the ciliary body:
> - T1: tumor limited to the ciliary body,
> - T2: tumor invading the AC and/or iris,
> - T3: tumor invading the choroidea,
> - T4: tumor with extra-scleral extension
>
> For choroideal melanomas:
> - T1: tumor ≤10mmn in its largest dimension with protrusion ≤3mm. T1a: tumor ≤7mm in its largest dimension with protrusion ≤2mm; T1b: tumor >7mm, but ≤10mm in its largest dimension with protrusion of >2mm and ≤3mm,
> - T2: tumor >10mm, but ≤15mm in its largest dimension with projection of >3mm and ≤5mm,
> - T3: tumor >15mm in its largest dimension with protrusion of >5mm,
> - T4: tumor with extra-scleral extension.

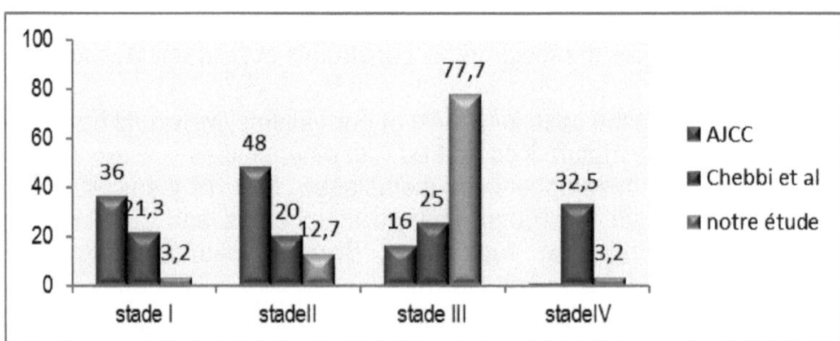

Fig. 44: Comparison of tumor classification between AJCC, Chebbi et al, and ours

4. Examens

4.1 OCT (optical coherence tomography) :

The main signs that can be studied on OCT are: maximum tumour thickness, rupture of Bruch's membrane, presence of orange pigments, existence of serous detachment of the neuroepithelium [62], Shields et al. [11] have described, within DSNE, a particular morphological characteristic of the photoreceptors called *shaggy photoreceptors*, hyper-reflective spots on the outer surface of the retina raised by the DSNE, in our study macular OCT was performed in 13 patients, a DSNE (serous detachment of the neuroepithelium) was found in half the cases, 38% had *shaggy photoreceptors* (N=13), Shields et al. [63], using EDI-OCT (Enhanced Depth Imaging Optical Coherence Tomography)in 37 patients with small choroidal melanomas, found *shaggy photoreceptors* in 49% of patients, and DSNE in 92% of cases (Fig. 45), *shaggy photoreceptors* correspond to hyper-reflective dots on the outer surface of the retina raised by the DSNE, overhanging certain melanomas. These dots, which are more or less elongated and sometimes ballooned, are present in 49% of melanomas, versus none in nevi [63].

Histologically, *shaggy photoreceptors* correspond to macrophage proliferations adherent to the posterior surface of the retina, containing melanin granules derived from the retinal PE [64]. These lesions are thought to exist in central serous chorioretinitis, choroidal hemangiomas and metastases, but their presence in suspected melanocytic lesions is almost pathognomonic for the diagnosis of melanoma [62].

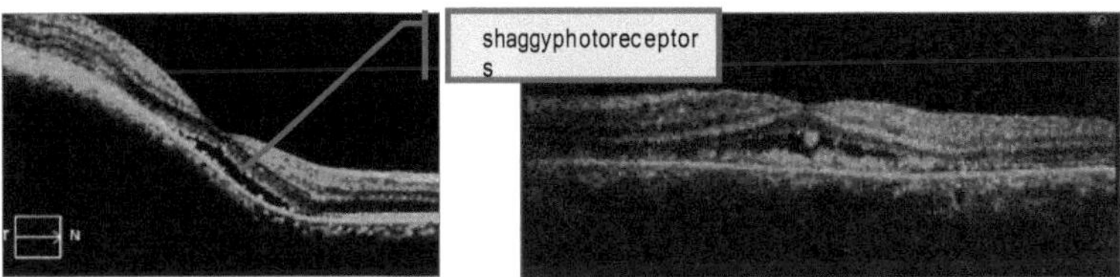

Fig. 45: Macular OCT, DSNE with shaggy photoreceptors, EHS ophthalmologie d'Oran

Chapter VII
Conclusion

Uveal melanoma is a rare cancer with a dismal prognosis, despite considerable advances in early diagnosis and quality of care in developed countries.
However, its annual incidence has been rising steadily over the past twenty years.

Our work was carried out in a referral center in western Algeria, and has resulted in sixty-three cases of uveal melanoma over a period of eighteen years, with an average of three cases diagnosed per year. The incidence of uveal melanoma in our population remains lower than that of the European population, but close to that of the Asian population of intermediate pigmentation.
On average, our patients are ten years younger at the time of diagnosis than the North American population. The wilayas most affected seem to be those in high latitudes.

At the end of our study period, we were able to make a number of sociodemographic and clinical observations on uveal melanoma in the Algerian context.
As for the clinical characteristics of neoformations, our tumors are thicker but less wide, with a high proportion of ruptures of Bruch's lamina, most often equatorial in location.

Our results seem to indicate an increase in uveal melanoma cases, but population-based multicenter observational studies are essential for a better appreciation of the incidence of uveal melanoma in the Algerian population.

Chapter VIII:
Bibliography

1.   A.Idder ; H.Yagoubi, M.A.Derdour A.Hadjari, A.Bekhti, H.Bénali, In 2014, uveal melanoma Etat des lieux à Oran Et Quoi de neuf? 17th Oran ophthalmology theme day, June 2014.

2.   N.Abi-Ayad, L .Kodjikian, J.Couturier Techniques for genomic analysis of uveal melanoma, 2011 JFO

3.   SFO Report: Intraocular tumors Leonidas Zografos 2002

4.   J Scotto, J F Fraumeni Jr, J A Lee ; Melanomas of the Eye and Other Noncutaneous Sites: Epidemiologic Aspects 1976

5.   Alsuhaibani AH , Uveal melanoma in the Saudi Arabian population: two decades of management at the King Khaled Eye Specialist Hospital, Saudi J.Ophthalmol 2009 Jul, Epub 2009 Aug 5

6.   Chebbi Amel, Bouguila Hedi, Alaya Nedia, Lejmi Houda, Malek Ines, Zeghal Imen, Nacef Leila ; Epidemiological aspects of uveal malignant melanoma in Tunisia. Department of ophthalmology, Hedi Raeis Institute. Tunis, LA TUNISIE MEDICALE - 2015

7.   Arun D. Singh, MD; Carol L. Shields, MD; Jerry A. Shields, MD; et alTakami Sato, MD ; Uveal melanoma in young patients, Arch Ophthalmol. 2000

8.   Singh AD, Topham A. Incidence of uveal melanoma in the United States: 1973-1997 Ophthalmology 2003

9.   Singh AD, Schoenfield LA, Bastian BC, Aziz HA, Marino MJ, Biscotti CV. Congenital uveal melanoma? Surv Ophthalmol 2016

10.   ShieldsCL, KalikiS, ArepalliS, AtalayHT, Manjandavida FP, Pieretti G et al. Uveal melanoma in children and teenagers. Saudi J Ophthalmol 2013

11.   Shields CL, Furuta M, Thangappan A, Nagori S, Mashayekhi A, Lally DR et al. Metastasis of uveal melanoma millimeter-by-millimeter in 8033 consecutive eyes. Arch Ophthalmol 2009

12.   Singh AD, Turell ME, Topham AK. Uveal melanoma: trends in incidence, treatment, and survival. Ophthalmology 2011

13.   Andreoli MT, Mieler WF, Leiderman YI. Epidemiological trends in uveal melanoma. Br J Ophthalmol 2015

14.   Park SJ, Oh CM, Kim BW, Woo SJ, Cho H, Park KH. Nationwide Incidence of Ocular Melanoma in South Korea by using the National Cancer Registry Database (1999-2011). Invest Ophthalmol Vis Sci 2015

15.   Biswas J, Kabra S, Krishnakumar S, Shanmugam MP. Clinical and histopathological characteristics of uveal melanoma in Asian Indians. A study of 103 patients. Indian J Ophthalmol 2004

16.   Phillpotts BA, Sanders RJ, Shields JA, Griffiths JD, Augsburger JA, Shields CL. Uveal melanomas in black patients: a case series and comparative review. J Natl Med Assoc 1995

17.   Hudson HL, Valluri S, Rao NA. Choroidal melanomas in Hispanic patients. Am J Ophthalmol 1994

18.   Windsor S. Davies, M.D. Detroit; Malignant melanomas of the choroid and ciliary body a clinicopathologic study, Michigan 1963

19.   Collaborative Ocular Melanoma Study Group Histopathologic Characteristics of Uveal Melanomas in Eyes Enucleated From the Collaborative Ocular Melanoma Study COMS Report No. 6

20.   Poso M.Y); Mwanza (J.C.K.); KAYEMBE (D.L.) ; Malignant tumors of the eye and adnexa in Congo-Kinshasa. JFO 2000

21.   Benjamin Miller, Cyril Abrahams, G. C. Cole, AND Neville S. F. Ocular malignant melanoma in South African blacks PROCTOR 1981

22.   M O Malik, E H El Sheikh ; Tumors of the eye and adnexa in the Sudan 1979

23.   P K Kuo, C A Puliafito, K M Wang, H S Liu, B F Wu; Uveal Melanoma in China 1970

24.   A. AZAK, M.D.; Cancer in Lebanon and the Near East 1962

25.   J W Harbour, M A Brantley Jr, H Hollingsworth, M Gordon ; Association between choroidal pigmentation and posterior uveal melanoma in a white populatio, Br J Ophthalmol 2004

26.   P K Kuo, C A Puliafito, K M Wang, H S Liu, B F Wu; Uveal Melanoma in China 1970

27.   Gonder et al uveal malignat melanoma associated with ocular and oculodermal melanocytosis, 1982

28.   Frederick C. Blodi, M.D; Ocular melanocytosis and melanoma 1975

29.   C L Shields [1], J A Shields, R C Eagle Jr, P De Potter, H Menduke; Uveal melanoma and pregnancy. A report of 16 cases 1991

30.   Johanna M. Seddon,' David T. Maclaughlin, 2 Daniel M. Albert,' Evangelos S. Gragoudas,' and Michael Ference; Uveal melanomas presenting during pregnancy and the investigation of estrogen receptors in melanomas III3, The British journal of ophthalmology 1982

31.   Jayne A. Buffey, Ian G. Rennie, Mark Benson, M. Andrew Parsons, Michael K. Faulkner, and Sheila MacNeil ; Effect of Melanocyte Stimulating Hormone on Human Cultured Choroidal Melanocytes, Uveal Melanoma Cells, and Retinal Epithelial Cells Tony Goodall 1994

32.   Cécile Laurent Thesis January 2011, Characterization of molecular markers associated with a high risk of developing metastases in patients with choroidal melanoma.

33.   Anne-Celine Derrien, MSc ,1, Manuel Rodrigues, MD, PhD,1,2, Alexandre Eeckhoutte, BSc ,1 Stephane Dayot, BSc ,1 Alexandre Houy, BSc ,1 Lenha Mobuchon, PhD ,1 Sophie Gardrat, MD,1,3 Delphine Lequin, MD,3 Stelly Ballet, MSc ,3 Gaelle Pierron, PhD ,3 Samar Alsafadi, PharmD, ,1,4 Odette Mariani, PhD ,5 Ahmed El-Marjou, PhD ,6 Alexandre Matet, MD, PhD ,7,8 Chrystelle Colas, MD, PhD,9 Nathalie Cassoux, MD, PhD,7,8 Marc-Henri Stern, MD, PhD ; Germline MBD4 Mutations and Predisposition to Uveal Melanoma 1,9,2020

34.   Michele Carbone, Haining Yang, Harvey I. Pass, Thomas Krausz, Joseph R. Giovanni Gaudino BAP1 and cancer University of Hawaii Cancer Center, 2014

35.   Manuel Rodrigues, Lenha Mobuchon, Alexandre Houy, Samar Alsafadi, Sylvain Baulande, Odette Mariani, Benjamin Marande, Khadija Ait Rais, Monique K. Van der Kooij, Ellen Kapiteijn, Sieta Gassama, Sophie Gardrat, RaymondL. Barnhill, Vincent Servois, Rémi Dendale, Marc Putterman, Sarah Tick, Sophie Piperno-Neumann, Nathalie Cassoux, Gaëlle Pierron, Joshua J. Waterfall, Sergio Roman-Roman, Pascale Mariani and Marc-Henri Stern ; Evolutionary Routes in Metastatic Uveal Melanomas Depend on *MBD4* Alterations Cancers 2021

36.   Ezekiel Weis, MD, MPH; Chirag P. Shah, MD, MPH; Martin Lajous, MD; Jerry A. Shields, MD; Carol L. Shields, MD; The Association Between Host Susceptibility Factors and Uveal MelanomaA Meta- analysis Arc Ophthalmol 2006

37.   Shah, Weis, Shield; Intermittent and chronic ultraviolet light exposure and uveal melanoma: à metanalysis. Ophthalmology 2005

38.   AndreaSchmidtPokrzywniakMA,PhD1KarlHeinzJöckelPhD2NorbertBornfeldMD3WolfgangSauer we [inMD4AndreasStangMPH, MD1Positive] Interaction Between Light Iris Color and Ultraviolet Radiation in Relation to the Risk of Uveal Melanoma: A Case-Control Study 2009

39.   P Guénel , L Laforest, D Cyr, J Févotte, S Sabroe, C Dufour, J M Lutz, E Lynge ; Occupational risk factors, ultraviolet radiation, and ocular melanoma: a case-control study in France 2001

40.   E A Holly , D A Aston, D K Ahn, A H Smith ; Intraocular melanoma linked to occupations and chemical exposures, , epidemiology Cambridge 1996

41.   Bruno F Fernandes, Jean-Claude A Marshall, Miguel N Burnier Jr; Blue Light Exposure and Uveal Melanoma, 2006

42.   Yi-Rui Ge, Nong Tian, Yan Lu, Yong Wu, Qin-Rui Hu, Zheng-Ping Huang; Occupational Cooking and Risk of Uveal Melanoma: a Metaanalysis 2012

43.   Daniel M. Albert, M.D., Carmen A. Puliafito, M.D., Anne B. Fulton, M.D., Nancy L. Robinson, A.B.,
Z. Nicholas Zakov, M.D., and Thaddeus P. Dryja, M.D
Increased incidence of choroidal malignant melanoma occurring in a single population of chemical workers 1980

44.   Ann Schalenbourg and Leonidas Zografos Bertil   Damato, Arun D. Singh Uveal Tumors Second Edition Clinical Ophthalmic Oncology 2014

45.   Demirci H, Shields CL, Shields JA, Honavar SG, Eagle RC Jr. Ring melanoma of the ciliary body: report on twenty-three patients. Retina 2002

46.   Hatem Krema, Bruno Fernandes, Rand Simpson, Hugh McGowan, Yeni H Yücel ; Knapp-Rønne choroidal melanoma: a clinicopathological report 2012

47.   Shields CL, Shields JA, De Potter P, et al.Arch Ophthalmol ; Diffuse choroidal melanoma. Clinical features predictive of metastasis. 1996.

48.   Reese AB, Howard GM. Am; Flat uveal melanomas. J Ophthalmol. 1967 Sayanagi K, Pelayes DE, Kaiser PK, Singh AD. 3D spectral domain optical coherence tomography fi ndings in choroidal tumors. Eur J Ophthalmol. 2011

49.   Smith LT, Irvine AR. Diagnostic signifi cance of orange pigment accumulation over choroidal tumors. Am J Ophthalmol. 1973

50.   Shields CL, Shields JA, Kiratli H, et al. Risk factors for growth and metastasis of small choroidal melanocytic lesions. Ophthalmology. 1995.

51.   Shields CL, Shields JA, Yarian DL, et al. Intracranial extension of choroidal melanoma via the optic nerve. Br J Ophthalmol. 1987

52.   Kuchle M, Nguyen NX, Naumann GO. Quantitative assessment of the blood-aqueous barrier in human eyes with malignant or benign uveal tumors. Am J Ophthalmol. 1994

53.   Castella AP, Bercher L, Zografos L, et al. Study of the blood-aqueous barrier in choroidal melanoma. Br J Ophthalmol. 1995

54.   Yap EY, Robertson DM, Buettner H. Scleritis as an initial manifestation of choroidal malignant melanoma. Ophthalmology. 1992

55.   Bujara K. Necrotic malignant melanomas of the choroid and ciliary body. A clinicopathological and statistical study. Graefes Arch Clin Exp Ophthalmol. 1982

56.   Biswas J, Ahuja VK, Shanmugam MP, et al. Malignant melanoma of the choroid presenting as orbital cellulitis: report of two cases with a review of the literature. Orbit. 1999

57.   KH Mesri, A.Derdour, S Nouasri, A.Idder; Massive extra scleral exteriorization of a uveal melanoma after phacoemulsification: about a case. SFO 2018

58.   Kivelä T, Summanen P. Retinoinvasive malignant melanoma of the uvea. Br J Ophthalmol. 1997

59.   O. Bergès, P. Koskas Échographie des tumeurs oculaires Fondation ophtalmologique Rothschild, PARIS. réalités ophtalmologiques # 214_June 2014

60.   Enrique Garcia-Valenzuela, MD, PhD; Chief Editor: Andrew A Dahl, MD, Choroidal Melanoma FACS, Feb 18, 2020

61.   J.F Korobelnik; OCT in ophthalmology, retinal and choroideal OCT, SFO2019.

62.   Carol L. Shields, MD; Swathi Kaliki, MD; Duangnate Rojanaporn, MD; Sandor R. Ferenczy, CRA; Jerry A. Shields, MD; Enhanced Depth Imaging Optical Coherence Tomography of Small Choroidal Melanoma Comparison With Choroidal Nevus, ARCH OPHTHALMOL / VOL 130 (NO. 7), JULY 2012

63.   Ralph C. Eagle Jr. Optical Coherence Tomography: Clinicopathologic Correlations -The 2016 Gordon K. Klintworth Lecture, Ocul Oncol Pathol 2018

64.   Pellegrini, Marco MD; Corvi, Federico MD; Invernizzi, Alessandro MD, Ravera, Vittoria MD; Cereda, Matteo G. MD; Staurenghi, Giovanni MD, FARVO; Swept-source optical coherence tomography angiography in choroidal melanoma An Analysis of 22 Consecutive Cases Author Information Retina: August 2019

65.   Zdravko Mandiæ, Jasna Talan-Hraniloviæ 2 De part ments of Oph thal mol ogy; 1Neurology; and 2Pathology ; Color Doppler Flow Imaging of Ocular Tumors Renata Ivekoviæ, Arijana Lovrenèiæ- Huzjan 1, Sis ters of Mercy Uni ver sity Hos pi tal, Zagreb, Croatia 2000

66.   Teresa A. Ferreira 1, Lorna Grech Fonk 1, Myriam G. Jaarsma-Coes Guido G. R. van Haren 1 Marina Marinkovic 2 and Jan-Willem M. Beenakker MRI of Uveal Melanoma 1,2, 17 March 2019

67.   Hakulinen T, Teppo L, Saxén E. Hakulinen Cancer of the eye, a review of trends and differentials. 1978

68.   J W Harbour, M A Brantley Jr, H Hollingsworth, M Gordon ; Association between choroidal pigmentation and posterior uveal melanoma in a white populatio, Br J Ophthalmol 2004

69.   Pradeep Manchegowdaa Arun D. Singhb Carol Shieldsc Swathi Kalikid Parag Shahe Lingam Gopalf Pukhraj Rishig, Uveal Melanoma in Asians: A Review, Ocul Oncol Pathol 2021

70.   Adel H. Alsuhaibani, Uveal melanoma in the Saudi Arabian population: Two decades of management at the King Khaled Eye Specialist Hospital, Saudi Journal of Ophthalmology 2009

71.   Diener-West M, Earle JD, Fine SL, Hawkins BS et al. Collaborative Ocular Melanoma Study Group. The COMS randomized trial of iodine 125 brachytherapy for choroidal melanoma, III: initial mortality findings. COMS Report no. 18. Arch Ophthalmol 2001

72.   Shields, C.L.; Kaliki, S.; Cohen, M.N.; Shields, P.W.; Furuta, M.; Shields, J.A. Prognosis of uveal melanoma based on race in 8100 patients: The 2015 Doyne Lecture. Eye 2015 Seddon, J.M.; Gragoudas, E.S.; Glynn, R.J.; Egan, K.M.; Albert, D.M.; Blitzer, P.H. Host factors, UV radiation, and risk of uveal melanoma. A case-control study. Arch. Ophthalmol. 1990

73.   Guénel, P, Laforest, L .; Cyr, D .; Févotte, J .; Sabroe, S.; Dufour, C.; Lutz, JM; Lynge, E. Occupational risk facts; ultraviolet radiation and ocular melanoma: a case-control study in France. Cancer Causes Control 2001

74.   Li, W.; Judge, H.; Gragoudas, E.S.; Seddon, J.M.; Egan, K.M. Patterns of tumor initiation in choroidal melanoma. Cancer Res. 2000

75.   Kaliki, S.; Shields, C.L. Uveal melanoma: Relatively rare but deadly cancer. Eye 2017

76.   Laurien E. Houtzagers, Annemijn P. A. Wierenga, Aleid A. M. Ruys, Gregorius P. M. Luyten and Martine J. Jager Iris Colour and the Risk of Developing Uveal Melanoma, September 28, 2020

77.   Frank G. AH-Fat, Bertil E. Damato Delays in the diagnosis of uveal melanoma and effect on treatment, Eye Royal College of Ophthalmologists 1998

78.   M Lahav, I Gutman, Am ; Subretinal pigment cells in malignant melanoma of the choroid J Ophthalmol 1978

79.   Proton therapy: cutting-edge technology at the interface between physics and medicine. 2011 Reflets de la physique n°26

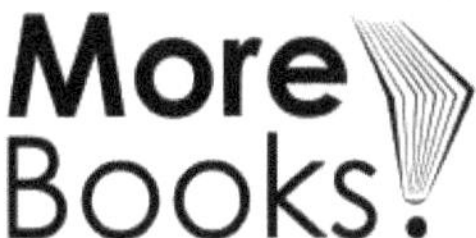

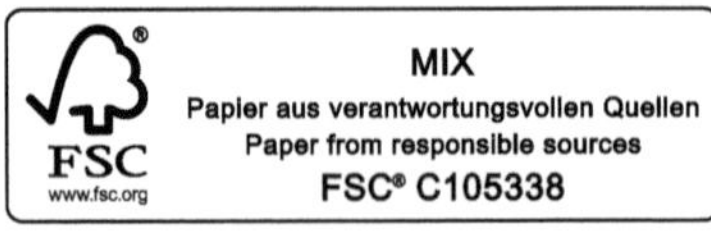

Printed by Books on Demand GmbH, Norderstedt / Germany